Reborn on the Run

Reborn on the Run

My Journey from Addiction to Ultramarathons

Catra Corbett
with Dan England

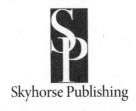

Skyhorse Publishing

Skyhorse Publishing books may be purchased in bulk at special discounts for sales promotion, corporate gifts, fund-raising, or educational purposes. Special editions can also be created to specifications. For details, contact the Special Sales Department, Skyhorse Publishing, 307 West 36th Street, 11th Floor, New York, NY 10018 or info@skyhorsepublishing.com.

Skyhorse® and Skyhorse Publishing® are registered trademarks of Skyhorse Publishing, Inc.®, a Delaware corporation.

Visit our website at www.skyhorsepublishing.com.

10 9 8 7 6 5 4 3 2

Library of Congress Cataloging-in-Publication Data is available on file.

Cover design by Tom Lau

Cover photo credit: Dan England

Print ISBN: 978-1-5107-2902-5

Ebook ISBN: 978-1-5107-2903-2

Printed in the United States of America.

Table of Contents

Chapter One

Blood, Blisters, and a Lot of Tears

The medic looked at my feet skeptically. My boyfriend blurted out the question that no one wanted to ask.

"You're done, right?" Kevin said to me.

The question pissed me off, but I couldn't blame him at the time for asking. I had just run sixty miles, ten miles longer than I had ever run in my life, and still I had forty more to go. No one, after seeing my feet, would advise me to go on. Hell, I knew that I probably shouldn't go on.

But I had to.

Kevin peered over the medic's shoulder as he peeled off my socks. Both of them gasped.

The balls of my feet were smothered in puffy half-dollars, my heels were completely blistered, and my toes had been overtaken by small pockets of white, painful bubbles. One of the half-dollars had already popped, leaking clear liquid steadily down my heel. The medic began to work on popping the other blisters while Kevin shook his head in disbelief.

This was my first hundred-mile race, and it was already clear I had a lot to learn. I'd made several mistakes. I was, for instance, nearly late to the race because of a last-minute dash to Walmart to buy a flashlight; it hadn't occurred to me that running a hundred miles would take all night.

And now I was suffering the consequences of my worst mistake. I was running the Rocky Raccoon 100 in Huntsville, Texas, a part of the country I knew nothing about. I lived in California, and I had no idea that the Texas humidity would make my feet swell the way a sponge expands after it soaks up water. I brought several pairs of socks—I knew you had to change them during a race—but I didn't know that I needed shoes a half-size larger than usual to make room for my ballooning feet.

California's dry air never gave me such problems. I'd never even had a blister before. Now my shoes were transforming my feet into tender-ized hamburger meat.

The medic scowled as he continued to work on my feet. Though ini-tially stunned by the blisters, he was a medic in an ultrarunning race, and he'd probably seen worse (at least, I hoped he had). I sighed with relief as fluid spilled out of the puffy pouches. He then started wrapping my feet in duct tape. Yes, the heavy-duty silver tape people used for household repairs, from leaky pipes to broken door handles. Until that moment I didn't know duct tape could also repair leaking blisters, but that was one of the many things I had yet to learn about being an ultrarunner. The tape secured the blisters against my skin, and when I got up to test them out, they felt pretty good for the first time in hours.

So no, Kevin, I wasn't done.

Like many people, I started running to get healthy. I switched all-night raves for early morning runs, and while I missed the rush of danc-ing till dawn, putting my sneakers away was not an option. I started like many do. I ran around the block, almost died, and then tried it again the next day and found I could go a little farther before I almost died again. I stumbled across ultramarathons just a few years after I became a runner. These impossibly-long races called to me. They seemed to be the answer I needed to change my life.

Four years after I started running, I competed in my first hundred-mile race. Just three months earlier I finished a fifty-miler, my second, in Napa Valley near my home in northern California, in pouring rain that left me soaked through and shivering but sure of my ability. I fin-ished last, but many ultrarunners much more experienced than me had dropped out of that race. I kept going. So I thought that if I could finish fifty miles, in those crappy, miserable conditions, while dodging or falling waist deep into muddy puddles, then I could run a hundred.

At least that's what I thought.

I picked the Rocky Raccoon randomly from the back of an ultrarunning magazine. This was 1999, and there were only a few hundred-mile races in the whole country (as of 2017, there are seventeen hundred-milers in California alone). I had lucked into a good one for beginners. Most of the race was in Huntsville State Park, just north of Houston. Five laps through the trees and swamps got you a hundred miles.

Beginners traditionally loved the course because it wasn't over mountains or hills, or even very rocky, despite the name of the race. Most of the trail was flat and wide, stuffed with soft dirt, making for a comfortable surface. It smelled like wood and mold and the air was heavy and wet, making it feel almost like a steamy sauna. The twenty-mile loop wound through scraggly woods that blotted out the sun, muddy swamps, and lakes full of creatures I'd never seen in California. A sign greeted you at the entrance: "Alligators Exist in the Park." Great.

Another reason beginners loved the trail were those laps. A huge aid station in a standalone tent, the kind you'd rent for a special occasion, greeted you at the end of every lap. There, runners could eat or drink, change shoes, put on or take off clothes, rub Vaseline on bloody friction rashes and, you know, have a medic put duct tape your battered, blistered feet.

As you entered, a sign warned that pukers should keep to the left. I was not a puker. At least, not yet I wasn't.

As I got up from my seat, stuffing my feet back into my too-tight shoes, the last rays of sunshine slipped behind the hills. In the thick cover of the trees, it was already dark. I would be running the rest of the race at night. I clicked my weak flashlight on and its beam danced around the trees like a pale strobe light. In a weird way, it reminded me of my old life—all that was missing was the deep beat of dance music reverberating in my chest.

"Good luck," the medic said, attempting to hide the worry in his eyes. "I hope the tape holds."

Why wouldn't the tape hold? Isn't that stuff used to repair just about anything?

Well, I'd find out soon enough. I started into my next lap.

Having laps is a little unusual for a long distance race. Many times, especially in an ultramarathon, you're stuck out there, alone, in the wilderness. You could get lost or thirsty or hurt, and no one would be around to help you for miles. That's why officials check you in when you make it to an aid station. If they don't cross your name off the list, they know they eventually have to start searching for you. Sometimes— especially if you look out of it—they ask you your name or weigh you to make sure you haven't lost too much weight.

But these were twenty-mile laps on the well-marked course with bright orange signs that you could see in the dark, which were like a security blanket for beginners like me. They meant that you were never too far from help, or a break, or water, before hitting the path for another twenty.

Still, no hundred miler is easy. The trail was clean but overrun with sneaky tree roots waiting to trip you if you weren't paying attention, and it's hard to pay attention for hours and hours of staring at the same damn trail. Your mind starts to wander, a kind of defense mechanism to stop you from thinking about the next mile, or the next forty. Spills, and the bloody knees and elbows they caused, were inevitable.

The duct tape padded my tender feet, and for the first time in a while, I felt better. I could run again. I was finally having fun. I wielded my flashlight and it gave off a sickly, yellow glow, but it was enough to let me see the roots and rocks so I wouldn't trip.

As the night settled around me, it muffled many of the sounds of the race through the forest. I heard the soft drumming of shoes on the dirt accompanied by a symphony of chirping crickets, croaking bullfrogs, and humming insects. The heavy breathing of other runners sounded like a breeze through the trees. Their conversations were hushed, as if no one wanted to disturb the calm of the night. "Good work," they said all around as they passed by.

A couple of runners trotted past me whispering encouragement to one another. I looked around noticing the huddles of runners packed together in small groups. Everyone but me seemed to have a buddy.

"They're called pacers," one runner said smiling as he passed by me. His pacer waved.

Pacers? You were allowed to have pacers? I had no idea, but yes, in hundred-mile races, you're allowed to have other runners with you on the course. Mostly what these people did was keep an eye on you and keep you from falling too deep into despair.

I'm all alone out here, I thought.

As the night closed in on me and the dark air constricted my breathing, the sounds of the race seemed to turn a bit more sinister. I thought back to that sign warning people who entered the park of alligators. In the dark, surrounded by the inky-black night, every time I heard something in the woods—a twig snapping or some underbrush rustling—my mind filled with snapping teeth.

That nervous energy carried me through the dark trail for a while and was enough to distract me from the steadily slipping duct tape flapping out of my sneakers.

Until it wasn't. Crap.

I really thought the duct tape would hold—if it fixed pipes, surely it could hold my feet together—but by mile seventy-five, the wet Texas air had once again soaked my feet with sweat. My shoes began to fill with needles, the pain from the blisters stabbing me with each step. It was some of the worst pain I'd ever felt.

And I still had a full marathon to go.

When I got into mile eighty, I collapsed in front of the same medic from before. He didn't exactly look psyched to see me.

"Let's take a look," he said, trying not to meet my eyes as I took off my shoes. It felt so good to get them off.

I didn't know anything about treating blisters, so I sat back in the chair, grimaced, and let him peel the tape off my heel. When he did, the skin slid off with it.

"FUUUUUUUUUUUUUCCKKKKKKKK," I screamed.

I braced myself as he took hold of the tape on my other heel. He pulled again and the skin came away as easily as if he was peeling an overripe banana. I screamed even louder this time. The raw patches burned and the warm midnight air offered no relief to the tender skin.

"I think you should stop," the medic said, finally looking me straight in the eye.

Even though I'd only completed a few races, I already knew that ultramarathons were as much about enduring as they were about running. There were others around me puking or cramping or hurting, or in various states of distress. So for him to tell me to quit was not only discouraging, it was frightening.

But fears be damned, I needed to finish this race. In my mind, I would not be an ultrarunner until I finished a hundred miler. I had finally found something that I thought could help me become a new person. It was the first thing in years that filled the void.

The medic's question scared me; but like Kevin's had before, it also pissed me off.

I stared defiantly back at him.

"Are you fucking kidding me?" I answered. "I came to run a fucking hundred miler. I'm not stopping now."

The medic sighed with resignation and started to cover my feet with fresh duct tape. I jammed my pathetic, swollen feet back into my shoes, which were nothing less than torture chambers at this point. As I stood up my legs quivered like a baby deer. I took a few steps, and it was the most excruciating pain I'd ever felt in my life.

Now my shoes felt like they were stuffed with hot coals. Tears ran down my face.

I took a few more steps and started into a slow jog. That pain would be with me for the next eight hours. It would be my pacer.

I had twenty miles to go, longer than most runners ever go in a single effort. Twenty miles is a half marathon, then a 10K, plus a mile, and I'd be doing it on feet that were as soft and sensitive as a baby's butt, on a trail riddled with tree roots and only the glow of my flashlight to show me the way. And then there were all those alligators that I was supposed to look out for.

It was pitch black now. The pain in my feet had reached fever pitch, but as I started yawning, it dawned on me that my feet weren't my biggest problem anymore.

I'd never run all night before, and I was yawning a lot now. A thick desire to curl up in the leaves and take a nap was threatening to end my race.

I couldn't take a break, no matter how badly I wanted one, because I was worried I wasn't going to finish before the cutoff time, when they pull runners off the course regardless of how far they've gone. Even the fastest runners can't afford to take much more than a catnap without missing the cutoff time, and I was one of the slowest. I had to keep going.

I weaved like a drunk driver across the wide trail, trying my best not to smash into other runners.

"Are you okay?" asked an older guy who'd obviously done this before. These types of guys always reminded me of my father. Later, many years after his heart gave out and he died when I was seventeen, I always thought my father would be one of those guys if his time wasn't cut short.

"I'm just so sleepy," I mumbled.

The guy nodded sympathetically. I wasn't the only one shuffling around like a zombie at this point.

"You need coffee," he said.

Coffee. Yes, I thought in a daze. *Yes. Coffee.* "Good luck!" he called over his shoulder as he jogged away into the darkness.

I was a couple miles from the next aid station. I knew if I could make it there, I'd be okay.

Coffee. Coffee. Coffee. It was a refrain I chanted with every painful step. All I wanted to do was lie down. I could barely hold my flashlight up, and its beam swung lazily across the trail, disorienting me. My eyelids slid closed while I continued to shuffle forward. They sprang open after I hit the ground with a thud. I pulled myself up brushing dirt from my hands.

Ultrarunners sometimes fall asleep on their feet because they're so tired. We can even doze off while we're running. I was lucky not to get hurt, but I was still exhausted as I stumbled forward. I was in serious trouble.

That's when I really felt the sense of community that led me to ultrarunning. Ultrarunners all look like regular people, the kind you might pass on a busy city street, but there's one key difference: they are all achieving these amazing physical feats. As other runners passed by and saw I was delirious from pain and exhaustion, something they'd felt themselves many times before, something many were feeling right now, they smiled and encouraged me, or asked if this was my first hundred miler (I'd hoped it wasn't that obvious, but I guess it was).

This was the kind of support I had been missing in my life since I had to move away from all my friends. Right then, my mom was the only one who seemed to be on my side. Even Kevin seemed to doubt me at times, as he did during this race.

But ultrarunners watch out for one another. It was as if everyone on that trail understood each other, and thus understood me, without evening knowing my story. A voice rang in my ears, out of the darkness.

"Can I get you anything?"

The aid station! I'd made it. Hell yes.

"I need coffee," I said.

"We don't have any," the volunteer said, her kindly face crinkling with sympathy.

My heart sank. I was done. I could run through pain, but I couldn't stay awake any longer.

"We could make some more," the volunteer said. "I think."

"How long will that take?" I said.

"Um . . . maybe twenty minutes or so?"

I didn't have twenty minutes. I'd stiffen up. My feet would turn into blocks. I'd probably fall asleep. My race was over. And then Kim's voice chirped behind me.

"Is this your first hundred? I haven't seen you before. I'm Kim," said a runner behind me in a warm Texas accent through bright-red lipstick. She obviously had done this race several times. "How are ya doin'?"

"I need coffee," I said back to her.

Kim shook her head. Her face was fully made up, which I thought was funny for a race. "You need NoDoz," she said. "Here, hon. I have some." She rummaged through a pack she wore and pulled out some small red pills.

A jolt of anxiety shot through me as she held them out to me. It was so tempting, but I knew I shouldn't. After all, I was out there almost dying while running a hundred miles because I was trying to ditch my life as a drug addict.

Patty, my oldest sister, was kind of mean. But Peggy was always nice to me, although she was bipolar and aloof. I was the youngest of the three girls in our family. Patty was nine years older than me, and Peggy was seven years older. We also had a brother, Jay, who was less than two years younger than me.

By the time Peggy was sixteen, she was frequently using drugs and drinking, probably because of her disorder. I was too young to realize it at the time—I was only nine years old—but she was already a drug addict.

Peggy was involved in all my earliest experiments with drinking and drugs. The first time I got drunk was at a Journey concert with her when I was only thirteen. Before I tried pot, she warned me: "If you're going to smoke pot, you have to be with me." It was her way of watching out for me.

Peggy would eventually develop a heroin addiction that put her on the streets, despite my mother's desperate efforts to save her. She just never found the thing that would help her forget drugs.

By the time my friends were pushing me to do meth, Peggy wasn't around to watch out for me. And as it turned out, without her, I had no barrier.

I had found a group of friends while working in a salon in my mid-twenties. We loved to go to Goth clubs and dance. They all did meth (speed) because it gave them the energy to dance. I always had the endurance to do that anyway—I would discover just how much I had later—but my friends all pushed me to try it anyhow. When I first saw it, it looked gross and scared me. That was enough to keep me away from it for a while. After many months of turning them away, I finally agreed to do it.

One night, a group of us were at a friend's house, waiting to go to a Goth club. I was with my boyfriend, Jason, who was in a band, which I thought was the coolest thing ever.

That night I wanted to stay up until sunrise at the club. I had trouble staying awake, but I loved dancing, and I loved the Goth scene. My friends talked about the magical energy meth gave you. The meth, I decided, would let me dance all night.

Everyone took a bump. Then it was my turn.

Jason handed me a clear ink pen that he had snapped in half and pointed to the line of white powder. It had a faint color, like yellow snow. My hands shook as I took the pen.

I snorted up the line, and it was just like huffing gunpowder through my nose.

The drugs rushed to the back of my throat, then dripped down, like I had an evil cold. It tasted like something you would use to strip paint. I grabbed a can of soda from Jason and guzzled it to try to wash away the revolting taste.

In a few minutes, my head melted into a warm, fuzzy, and buzzing energy. It was like I was looking at the world from the window of a moving subway, only I had the energy to keep up with it.

I didn't like the buzzing. It made my head feel like a bug zapper. But I loved the energy. I loved that I could dance all night without feeling tired. I felt unstoppable.

After that night, for six months, we used meth as a booster and nothing more. It was a fun, recreational drug. When you snorted it, it felt like drinking five cups of coffee, one after another. We'd snort it when we wanted to drive to LA, a few hours away, to go to the clubs. The drug always gave us the energy to stay up all night. It seemed like a miracle drug, really.

You'd pay a price for it though. Coming down from that high felt like the flu, an illness that would not allow me to sleep. It felt like my brain was rubbing against exposed wires. I was starving and yet nothing sounded appetizing.

I could avoid that, for the most part, by sleeping it off. I was usually so tired by then, anyway, that I could sleep for twelve hours or longer, and when I'd wake up, I'd feel good again.

But one night in 1991, I was coming down from a night of snorting meth, and I had Lollapalooza to go to the next day.

Now, every addict has a defining moment, and mine was then. Lollapalooza featured a dream bill of punk, alternative, dance, electronic, and metal. It was a sensation and was right up my alley. I was supposed to go with a really good friend. I didn't want to miss it.

But I was also in the throes of that same, crappy, crackling flu, and the friend suggested that I take more.

"If you do speed now," she told me, "you'll feel better."

It sounded disgusting, like the way a martini sounds after a hangover, but I didn't want to miss the show. I snorted more meth, gagging at that same metallic taste, but after a few minutes, I did indeed feel better. And I realized then that I didn't need to suffer the effects of a comedown. And that's the day that meth stopped being a recreational drug. It was a drug

I took to feel normal. I'd never have to feel bad again. I'd just do more meth. I thought I'd found the solution to avoiding the lows.

I was so wrong.

Two years later, I hated my life. When you're an addict, the drugs no longer give you that awesome energy. They suck it out of you. The only reason that you keep on doing them is because it's so much worse when you don't.

I managed to hold down my job at the hair salon, but I was avoiding my family.

I had always been close to my parents, but when I was hooked, I saw my mother maybe once a month. I was ashamed of what I'd become. Peggy had already disappointed her so many times. And that's what I was doing then, too. Countless times, I'd make plans to see Mom, with good intentions, but I wouldn't show up.

After a while, when the drugs no longer gave me the energy I craved, meth painted my world in a curtain of grey. It was dull and lifeless and hopeless.

Those rare times I was sober, the curtains parted and the world returned to me, and I would stare out of my car window and be amazed at how colorful everything was, how bright and vibrant and alive it all seemed.

My life sucked. The drugs were all I had.

I couldn't dance at the clubs any longer, or hang out with my friends, or be a good daughter or sister. I didn't want to be the person I'd become, but I didn't know how to change. And then the cops broke down my door.

I looked down at the small caffeine pill in my hand. I now knew that there can actually be two defining moments in an addict's life: when you get hooked, and, if you're lucky and determined, when you decide to quit. The night in jail after the police broke down my door scared me so much, I knew I had to quit.

I'd done well up until that point to stay off drugs—I moved away from my friends, stopped going to the clubs, and had given up alcohol.

I stayed true to my diversion program and went to NA meetings every day. I was working in a bagel shop. But it was hard. I missed my friends, the deafening music of the clubs, and the rush from a bump of speed, especially now as I faced that last twenty miles.

I didn't want to take anything that even resembled drugs. I was out there running to forget them. I was hoping ultrarunning would be the thing that would help me forget drugs. I was hoping ultrarunning would be the one thing that Peggy never had. And so any kind of drugs made me nervous after my addiction. I didn't even take Advil any more, despite, you know, the fact that pain meds can really help you through a hundred-mile race.

I rolled the tiny caffeine pill around in my hand. It seemed a lot like the speed that kept me awake for hours on end in my old days. It would give me the same kind of energy. As badly as I needed it, this scared the shit out of me.

"It's just like coffee," Kim said, sensing my hesitation. "It's the exact same amount of caffeine."

She could see that I was still worried.

"Just take half," she said.

I popped the pill into my mouth, bit it in half, and tucked half away. Just fifteen minutes later, I was awake.

The other runners all seemed to be out there to cheer me on. It was the kind of support that was, well, addicting. I started on again, following Kim until she ran ahead. I felt better knowing that she and her red lipstick smile would be out there on the course with me.

As I started into the last twenty miles, my feet begged me to stop. I walked and ran through the heat of my chaffing toes and the cold of my shredded heels. The haze of my exhaustion and the buzz of the caffeine was all that kept me going. It really was like a dream. A nightmare really. Only my tears and the stabbing pain reminded me that I was still out there, on the course, trying to be an ultrarunner.

The sounds of the night, the buzzing bugs, and the whispers of the other runners all faded as the first light washed through the trees. The thick branches blocked most of the early morning light. The dim light made things seem that much more surreal. I would see a tree or a bush and think it was another runner. The tree roots on the ground turned to snakes slithering from the swamp. I jumped out of range of imaginary fangs a few times, yelping when I landed hard on my ruined feet.

I was miserable, in a painful daze. I kept going, but doubts were just behind me, on my heels, while the pain continued to pace me.

I began to yawn again—the NoDoz was just starting to wear off. The crickets were silent, but I could hear birds chirping. I could see the sky begin to glow, and I stashed my flashlight.

As I ran out of the trees, the morning sunlight washed over me. It was warm and bright, and energy spread through me. The birds grew louder. The crowd was bigger. The end was closer.

My head was full of thoughts of my dad as I stumbled through those last few miles. I talked to my father in my head with pride. *Look at what I'm doing now, Dad*, I said to him as I stumbled home, bawling.

Just get there, I thought. *Just a few more miles. Just get there.*

The faint cheering that had teased those last few miles slowly became louder, and I ran a little faster.

My feet hurt and my legs were killing me, but they worked. I thought of my dad, of Peggy, of all the addicts I had left behind, the runners whose bodies were too broken to run again. I was running for all those who couldn't.

I rounded a corner, one that I'd seen four times. The cheering got even louder. I realized I had less than a mile go to, and then I saw the finish.

When I finally crossed the finish line in that mad dash, I thought a bolt of lightning would strike me down. Or something corny like that. But it wasn't nearly as dramatic. I crossed the line, kicked off my shoes and the duct tape hanging from my battered feet, and fell to the floor smiling.

I never did see any alligators.

Back in the hotel room after a hot bath and a quick trip back to the race course because I forgot the buckle they give you for running a hundred miles, I called Jim Boyd.

Jim, whom I called Jimbo, was one of those older guys who reminded me of my father. I met him while running a trail marathon. It was our first trail marathon, and we both got lost and found our way back together. He was the first example of the kindness and camaraderie I discovered in the ultrarunning community.

We were supposed to run Rocky Raccoon together, but he had gotten injured.

"I finished," I told him, enthusiastically.

"Great! Good job, Catra!" his warm voice filled me with pride. "So what about doing that twenty-four-hour race I talked about?"

Jim had told me about this race about a week before. The entire gist of it was to run as far as you could in twenty-four hours. Maybe I could break a hundred miles in twenty-four hours if it was on a track and I had shoes that were a half size bigger.

I looked down at my raw bleeding feet. My body hurt more than it had ever hurt in my life. I honestly didn't know how long it would take me to walk again. All I wanted was to sleep, but the memory of crossing that finish line lingered in my mind.

I smiled. *Why not?*

When you're trying to quit something as all-consuming as drugs, you need to find something else you're passionate about. You have to find something else that will help you feel good. The addicts at the meetings volunteered, or helped others, or found a good job. I never found that thing that could help me quit.

I had finally found my thing that would keep me off drugs. It was a painful passion, for sure, but going off drugs was painful too.

I was now an ultrarunner.

Chapter Two

One Night in Jail Makes a Hard Woman Crumble

Before I was an ultrarunner, I was a drug addict. I was a hair stylist, and a go-go dancer on the weekends, and a daughter and a girlfriend and a friend to many, but I was mostly a drug addict. And by that, I mean that everything I did, I did to get high.

At the time, I was working at a hair salon, and it was a great job. I was making a lot of money. I could work twelve-hour days, no problem, because in between clients, I would go to the bathroom and snort meth.

I enjoyed my days working in the salon. It was creative work and it matched my love for clothes and doing my hair in all these crazy ways; plus it let me get high. I was always high.

And the meth gave me the energy to do other things as well.

On the weekends, I loved to dance. That dancing was the only work-out I had then. At the time, I hated running and wouldn't go near the gym. So dancing was a way to stay fit. I loved going out to clubs and dancing anyway, so I made some extra money working as a go-go dancer. I wore only a bra and a G-string, but I didn't care because I was high. I never really got the whole appeal of guys just standing there, watching them and watching me, and giving all of us money. Honestly, it was a creepy place to make money. But I made good money there and, honestly, I didn't care. I was high.

The whole idea was to make a bunch of money so we could go buy more drugs and sell more drugs so we could do more drugs. My boyfriend, Jason, sold most of the drugs, but I helped him sell more.

So I worked and danced. I could work all day and then I could dance all night. I had a lot of energy. I felt great. I felt euphoric. I felt high. I could accomplish a lot on drugs.

Until you had to come off them.

When you are on drugs, you live in a haze, a bubble of sorts, and you are left aware of only yourself and a few people around you. There was a steady supply of drugs because Jason and I were small-time dealers, so I had it around all of the time. But when I didn't have it, and the drugs wore off, my mind was no longer just hazy. It was really foggy. I was a mess.

Life caught up with me then. The things that made me tired, such as staying up for three days straight or working twelve hours a day or dancing all night, suddenly made me exhausted. That amazing, intense feeling was replaced by a thin shade of gray. The wonder of life was gone.

I would sleep for two days straight sometimes when I was off drugs.

I hated that feeling.

So I was rarely off drugs.

So I felt great most of the time. Because I was high.

But the drugs began to eat at me.

I was living with Jason at his parent's house at the time. It was nice living with a family. His parents were really kind and cared about me. But, like many families, it was also messed up. Jason's brother would stumble home wasted almost every night, and every weekend his parents would sit around and get drunk and argue.

I rarely saw my own family then. I did my mother's hair once a month, and she would suggest that we go to lunch. I would agree to it, and then I would either forget about it, or more often, I just wouldn't show up. I didn't want her asking questions about my life. I didn't want her to know anything about me, about who I'd become. I was ashamed of who I was, even when I was having fun doing it.

Like most addicts, I started losing stuff when I was on drugs. My car was repossessed, and that's not because I didn't have the money: I just wasn't paying bills. I would just forget to. I was forgetting about more and more things that one needed to do to be a normal, functioning adult in society. My friends and I had our own society. We got high and danced.

So we had money, but other than buying drugs to take away the pain of coming down, we couldn't enjoy what we'd worked so hard to earn. We essentially had no life. We didn't have our own place, and we drove a shitty, crappy car with no heater. At night, even though we lived in California, it would be freezing. I was dressed scantily to go to the club, and I'd have to bring blankets to wrap around my body.

I was also snorting several times a day, and it got to the point where I didn't know how much I was doing. I was out of control.

I started losing stuff.

I started losing friends and family.

I started losing myself. It was bad.

This last statement was, in fact, doubly true. I wasn't eating, and when I was eating, the drugs seemed to melt my weight away. I was already thin, but my friends and I became fascinated with how much weight we were losing. We would weigh ourselves many times a day and would be amazed by the results: "Wow! Look! Ninety-eight pounds!" I became obsessed with it. As a result, I developed an eating disorder that would haunt me for years later, even as I began to get into ultrarunning.

But the drugs just didn't eat away at my weight; they also whittled away at my sanity. I began to feel paranoid. When Jason went out at night, if I decided to stay home, I would constantly peek out of the window and see people who weren't there staring at me across the street with green eyes. I would hear things. I would hear voices. I was convinced that Jason's cat was trying to kill me.

My friends were doing drugs as hard as I was, and the drugs started to eat at them too. One friend would lock himself inside because he was afraid of the outside world. (I was reminded of this friend again when I was running ultramarathons when other runners nearing seventy-five miles or so would startle late at night, convinced they had just seen a demon on the dark trail, and scream or run faster or cover their faces. I would just laugh, because I knew they were hallucinating.)

So I would do more drugs to quiet the voices in my head, and make the people across the street disappear, and make those hallucinations go away. I was barely living.

I found needles and soon discovered that Jason was shooting meth. I could already tell he was getting really bad, and I had friends who had told me the same thing. When I asked him, though, he would lie to me and tell me that they were his friends' needles. So I would ask Jason about it, and he would lie, but I didn't really want to confront him about it. I was addicted, too, and so I honestly didn't care. I was into my own addiction. I didn't care about anything except getting high. I snorted and worked and snorted and danced and helped Jason sell drugs and snorted.

This was serious. Shooting drugs is usually the last step before addicts either get arrested, die, or get so hooked that would eventually wind up on the street and disappear.

One day, I looked at myself in the mirror, and I felt like shit and needed to do more drugs, and it hit me: I realized that this was my life. I was doing everything for drugs. It wasn't for love or for my parents or for myself. It was for the drugs.

But I saw no way out. I thought this sucks, but it's also who I am. This is who I'm going to be. I saw no way to change that.

And then I got high.

That day, or maybe it was just a day later, a friend called me up. I picked up the phone, and I set a deal to sell him some drugs.

I found out later that he had gotten arrested earlier in the day, and the cops found some speed on him, and they were asking him who his main dealers were. They wanted to get the "big guys." Our friend told the cops that he got the drugs from us.

But our friend hadn't gotten them from me or Jason this time, even though we did occasionally sell him drugs. On this particular incident he bought them from another guy, a guy way above us; but he wasn't going to turn that guy in because who knows what would have happened if he had turned him in? He probably would have killed our friend and us too.

When our friend called me, the cops were on the other end of the phone, coaching him on what to say. I never thought that was even possible. Hell, I'd never even been arrested.

Two days later, I was in the kitchen with some of Jason's family, heating up food, when someone starting thumping on the door.

"Open up! This is the police!" *Oh, shit.*

"Who is Catra? Who is Jason?" the cops yelled, barging in.

They held everyone on the ground. Jason's parents, brother, and his brother's girlfriend were all looking at me.

I told them I was Catra.

The police started raiding the house. They asked us if we had any weapons and where our drugs were.

His parents kept asking what was going on while the cops stormed through.

Things settled down a bit once the cops began to realize that we weren't that big-time dealers. We were cooperating and showing them where the drugs were, and we didn't have any illegal guns. They soon stopped searching the house, and they realized that Jason's parents had nothing to do with it.

Then a cop sat me down and told me Jason and I were going to jail.

A policeman who took me to the car was really nice. He could tell that I was scared because I was crying and frantic and shaking. He sat me in the back of the car and began to talk to me.

"Why are you involved with this guy?" he asked. I couldn't answer.

"You look like a good person. You've never been in trouble. Why?" I couldn't answer.

I knew it was because I had to get high.

He told me it would be OK, and that I would probably be out on bail the next day, and that he would make sure I was in my own cell. But he also said that I would be going to jail.

We rode and wound up in downtown San Jose, handcuffed, and they brought us into an interrogation room.

At the station, Jason took the blame, and they separated us. He stayed there, and they took me to a women's correctional facility.

The first place I went actually reminded me of a waiting room or an airport terminal. There were magazines lying around and there was even a small TV. But I was terrified. The only thing that kept me going was knowing that I would probably be released soon and that if I was going to be in jail for a couple hours, that I would be in my own cell.

There were other women around, and we all began talking to each other. Some of us looked like we should be there, but most of us didn't. The one person who really stood out to me was this older woman who looked like a grandmother. The poor woman had simply gotten into an argument with her husband, and when the police came, they discovered scratch marks on him. She was arrested for spousal abuse.

But soon the police came and took me in a back room and strip searched me, and then they gave me a jumpsuit that made me look like a big, orange carrot.

I was so skinny and small at the time that the clothing was just falling off me.

The officer then told me I would be staying the night there.

"Wait," I said. "One of your guys told me I'm not supposed to be here. I'm not supposed to be here. I'm not supposed to be here!"

But they laughed at me and brought me into the main part of the jail.

"Guys, I'm really, really not supposed to be here."

"I'm really, really not supposed to be here." I said this probably twenty times, over and over, but as they led me to the cell, with many other woman, it occurred to me that maybe I was supposed to be there. Reality started to sink in, and I became really, really scared.

I'm going to jail, and I'm going to stay the night with all these other people who do criminal activity, I thought. *I'm not a criminal.*

But of course I was. Even though I didn't think I was hurting people, I was doing something illegal. I had done it all along. I was even hurting people I loved, but I just didn't realize it because I was so into my own addiction.

I was handed a toothbrush, comb, and wooly blanket. I especially hated the feel of the blanket. It felt very scratchy, and there was something about it. It felt gross and awful and used and very, very unsettling. Later, whenever I would finish a long race and was shivering, even with hypothermia, if they put one of those wool blankets over me, I would yell at the person to get it off me.

In the cell, there was a stainless steel mirror, and I could see myself with the awful wool blanket and the orange clothes. I asked myself what the policeman asked me earlier.

What was I doing here?

This is not me, I thought. *I really wasn't a bad person, like the policeman said. And I didn't want to be there any longer.* Something had to change.

The next morning, after a sleepless, scared night with all the other criminals, I was sitting with these women at breakfast, picking at a crappy sandwich and some fruit and juice. Someone wanted my sandwich, so I gave it to her, and then I told them that I was leaving today.

"Oh, you're not getting out of here," one of the women said. "They never let people out on a Saturday. You're not going to court until Monday."

My heart sank, and I got more scared. I started crying again. I was so full of despair. I didn't want to be in there, and I didn't want to be around those people any longer, and I didn't want to be around myself, either. I felt like a criminal. I didn't like that feeling.

And then I heard my name being called.

I was getting out.

I was so relieved.

And though I didn't realize it at the time, I had just taken my first step to getting off drugs.

When my court process started, my attorney was pushing for no jail time. He told the court I had a job and that I would go through an outpatient program. The judge agreed and obliged me to undergo a diversion program.

The program meant that if I went through treatment, passed all the weekly drug tests, and the drug testing program, then the charges would be dropped.

When I started to go to the drug diversion meetings, I was a little amazed at how many people were still doing drugs. I would go to meetings, and in between the talks, people asked me how I was getting away with the pee tests. There were all kinds of ways to mask your pee, and they would all compare what they were using.

I told them I wasn't on drugs. I told them I was just peeing. They all acted surprised.

When I would sit in the meetings, I slowly began to realize that these people all had stories. They had seen a lot of crazy shit. They had seen people die, even close friends or family. Some of them, even the women, were gang members. They had spent time in prison.

I would just sit back and listen to what they had to say. They didn't like that I was quiet. They would ask me to contribute more, but I didn't have a lifetime of stories like they did. I would explain that their stories were a lot more amazing than mine. They had a lot more to say than I did.

After six months of those meetings and Narcotics Anonymous, I wasn't obligated to go to the meetings, but I went anyway. I went for another six months, but soon started to think the meetings weren't for me. All members did was talk about the past. I wanted to move forward. I wanted to focus on the future. I didn't feel the need to keep rehashing things over and over again.

After our arrests, Jason and I weren't doing well as a couple, but I still lived with him and his parents.

I would still try to see my friends in the nightclubs and go out with them, but they would all smoke and drink. The nightclubs didn't have the same feel that it once did. It didn't have the same allure. Even the music sounded different. It didn't bring me any joy. Before, hearing music always made me want to move and dance and have fun, but now it sounded lifeless to me.

I just felt sad for everyone there. I felt like they were covering or hiding something by drinking or doing drugs. They were still losing who they were.

I didn't feel better than them. In fact, in some ways, I wasn't nearly as happy as they were. I was depressed and felt out of place, like I didn't really know who I was or what I was doing. But I began to feel like I was finding myself too.

I just didn't want to be a part of the scene any longer.

My therapist was really helping me dig into my life and figure out what I was trying to cover up with the drugs. We called that "medicating" in the drug world, and it turned out there was more than I thought. I'd had some bad shit happen to me when I was young. I needed to work through those issues.

I was still working at a hair salon, part-time, but getting off the drugs and leaving them and my friends made me sadder than I'd ever been in my life. It was ironic, but I was becoming way sadder than that day I stared at myself in the mirror and thought there was no way out of being an addict.

I wasn't happy with Jason, and I wasn't happy being around my friends, and one of the few things I really loved to do, dance at the nightclubs, didn't bring me any joy either. My whole life just really, really sucked. I felt nothing, like I was in this big, deep black hole, and it was becoming darker.

One day, I just decided I didn't want to be here any longer. I was off drugs, but I hated myself for what I'd become, still, and I wanted it to be over.

I didn't have a gun, and I wasn't going to stab myself, but something popped into my head. *Tylenol.*

I put as many as I could into my hand and swallowed as many as I could. I began crying, and I took more and more, forcing myself to swallow the pills through my sobbing. Finally I lay down on the bed I shared with Jason and tried to cry myself to sleep, with the intent of never waking up again.

And then a little voice began to speak to me.

"You are better than this," it told me. "You will become someone."

I don't know why I listened to it, as depressed as I was, but I did.

I jumped up, called 911, and told them what I did. They came and rushed me to the hospital in an ambulance, and then they pumped my stomach.

It was, probably, the worst thing I've ever experienced.

They stuck a tube down my throat and made me gag and gag and gag up everything in my stomach. I couldn't stop. It was so awful.

I stayed in the psych ward that night. I was released the next morning after meeting with my therapist, even though you are supposed to stay there for seventy-two hours. The doctors didn't think I really wanted to kill myself, even though I had tried. I met with my therapist, and she told me that I needed to get out of Jason's house, since it was a really unsafe place for me.

I had to promise that I would leave there as soon as I could, and when I did that, I was let go.

I knew I would have to call my mother and tell her what had happened with my life.

My hands shook as I picked up the phone. I didn't want to tell my mother that I was on drugs. I knew it would break her heart.

A daughter calling to say that she was addicted to drugs would probably break any mother's heart, but I knew it would devastate her because of Peggy.

My sister Peggy was a drug addict from the time she was fifteen. When Peggy got hooked, my mother devoted much of her life trying to cure her. It was, in many ways, her mission in life.

My parents really did love her, and it broke their hearts to have so much trouble with her.

By the time I made that phone call, my mother had spent decades with Peggy's addiction haunting her. She spent tens of thousands of dollars trying to help Peggy beat her addiction to heroin, but the hard truth was, Peggy didn't really seem to want the help. My mother never really seemed to realize it. She put Peggy in clinics and treatment centers, and it never worked.

The sad thing was, at times, Peggy did seem to want to get better. In fact, there was a time when she was a normal person, not an addict. Peggy got married at eighteen and had a couple kids and seemed to be doing fine. But she was not fine. She never did kick her addiction. She just set it aside for a while.

Three years later, at age twenty-one, Peggy met up with her high school sweetheart, and just like that, she went back to her old ways. Her demons called her back into the flock. She left her family and became homeless. At this point, my mother not only spent money, she spent hours driving around with a friend on the streets of San Francisco, looking for Peggy on the street, hoping to scoop her up and save her.

At this point, my mother heard from Peggy only occasionally. Peggy would come by whenever she needed a few bucks. She would say she needed money for cigarettes, and you would say that you would go to the store to get them, but she didn't want any part of that. She wanted the money.

She wanted money for drugs. My mother knew that much at least. She refused to give her money. She couldn't even leave her purse lying around when Peggy came over because the money would go missing, and then Peggy wouldn't even believe that she stole it from her. She wouldn't remember taking it.

She was that bad. She was that out of it. She was that into her drugs.

Patty and I wondered at this point when the police would show up at my mother's door and tell us Peggy was dead. My mother refused to believe it could ever happen. She always hoped Peggy could get better.

Still, my mother was not naïve. She knew what heroin could do to someone, and after seeing what it did to Peggy, I knew she would refuse to believe that anyone else could fall for it. She would refuse to believe, for instance, that I had become an addict as well.

Peggy tried to warn my mother about me. She told her occasionally that she thought I was on drugs because I was so thin and because of the way I dressed. But my mother never believed her.

I never really believed it either. I wasn't a drug addict because I wasn't sticking a needle in my arm like Peggy. Peggy was the addict. I wasn't an addict. A night in jail changed my thinking.

Now I'd have to admit, once again, to my mother, and to myself, that I was an addict.

"Hello?" my mother answered.

I took a deep breath.

"I want to move back home," I said.

"That's fine," my mother said. "What's up?"

"Well," I said, "I was arrested."

"What?"

"Um, it was for selling drugs."

"What?" Louder.

I tried to dull the blow a bit. "We did speed once in a while. So we started selling to pay for it."

"WHAT?" Screaming.

There was a pause. I could tell that she was disappointed, and she was also angry, which was hard to hear.

"Catra, you should know better," my mother finally said. "Your sister is a drug addict."

I didn't know what else to say to her. She was right, but I also thought it was strange that she thought I should just know not to do drugs because my sister was an addict.

"I just want you to know that I'm going to move back home, and that I was in an outpatient program and that I had to go to meetings and that I am getting better," I told her.

My mother was silent. She said when I moved in that I would have to sit down with her and tell exactly her what happened.

A few days later, Jason's parents dropped me off. They said hi to my mother, but she didn't say much. My mother didn't like them. She didn't think they were a good influence. She was probably right.

When we got back to her house, she told me to sit down, like I was a little girl.

I sat at the table. It reminded me of growing up Catholic.

When I was a little girl, I'd have to go to church. I loved the stained glass windows and all the statues, but at the same time, I hated the old, scary building. It smelled stale. Most of all, I hated going into the confession booth because it always freaked me out. The priest slid open that little window and you had to tell him your sins. It was a dark little box, and he would talk on the other side and listen as you told him your darkest secrets and waited for your punishment.

Sitting across from my mother, I felt like that kid again in that dark little box, scared to tell someone the truth and hoping that I wouldn't go to hell.

I took another deep breathe, and I told her everything. I told her I'd been doing drugs for a few years.

"WHY?" she answered.

She didn't want to listen.

"You should KNOW better," she said, over and over.

She was angry and looking back, I can't blame her. The last thing she needed, and thought she would have to deal with, was another daughter on drugs. She had enough horrible memories of doing shit like driving the streets of San Francisco late at night looking for my sister.

Then she brought up Peggy again.

"You know, Peggy told me that she thought you were on drugs," my mother said, "but I didn't listen to her because she's a drug addict, and she doesn't know what she was talking about. But she wasn't lying or wrong. For once, she wasn't lying."

So I just told her that I had lost my way. She really didn't want to hear more than that.

I moved in, and I had to go by her rules, basically. She wanted to make sure I wouldn't be like my sister, going in and out of programs.

Moving in with my mother back in Fremont was depressing for me. Before I moved in, I thought I was doing pretty well. I was living on my own, I was making a bunch of money, and I could do whatever I wanted and had my own life.

But it wasn't a life for me. It was a life for drugs. Yes, I was making money, but that money went towards drugs. Yes, I was living on my own, but it was with Jason and his fucked-up family.

I was going to meetings and doing drug tests and working, and I was very embarrassed about who I had become. I had lost my way. I was so sad and felt like I had let my mother down.

Ultimately, I wanted all the gross drugs out of my life. I wanted to become a new person. Maybe it would be the person I should have been a while ago. It was the person I think my Dad would want me to be.

So I began running.

Chapter Three

Daddy's Girl

One of my first childhood memories is of the races my father would orchestrate between my brother and me.

Dad would take us outside because my mother used to clean our house on Sundays. So my father would take us to a high school football field and would stand in the middle of it while having us do these relays where we had to run back and forth.

I hated every second of it.

I was such a girly girl that when I played outside, I would cry if I got dirty.

So I obviously hated racing my brother. I would push as hard as I could, but my brother would always kick my ass. It only made it worse that he was about two years younger than me and still always beat me.

"You're doing great, peanut," Dad would yell. "Just push as hard as you can."

A couple years later, when I was seven and my brother was five, my parents decided that they would sign us both up for soccer.

But I didn't want to play soccer. I loved to tap dance. I would even sleep with my tap shoes on. I would get so excited. I loved the clicking of the shoes. I loved the outfits. When you practiced for several months, you would get to perform in a show, and that meant you got to wear makeup and do your hair up and wear sparkling clothes, things you never got to do when you were only seven. I was fascinated with glamour. I would watch *Soul Train*, the TV show with all the black dancers moving to funk, because of all the fancy outfits they would wear. I just loved all of it.

My father became the coach for my brother's team and decided to be the coach for my team as well. But I was not a good team player. I would sit on the sideline while the others ran up and down the field. I was afraid to get dirty and I would protest saying I didn't want to do it. Eventually I did what he told us to do, but I hated it. I hated the running.

Because of where my birthday fell in the year, I was always the youngest on the team. I was eleven, for instance, but I wound up on a twelve and older team. When I was thirteen, it seemed like all the girls were fourteen and fifteen. So they were all older and bigger, and I always felt a lot smaller and weaker.

Around the same time, my dad also enrolled me in a softball league, and we would practice in the backyard. One day the sun was in my face, and the ball hit me in the nose because I couldn't see it.

After that, I was terrified and screaming bloody murder at the ball and became afraid of balls in general. During soccer, I would just turn my back whenever the ball came toward me. I began to hate sports in general.

Dad continued to try to connect with me through sports. It would take me years, many years after he was gone, to realize how much he influenced me.

One day while I was a preteen, when I walked into the family room, hoping my parents wouldn't talk to me, there was a program on about the Western States 100, the most prestigious ultramarathon in the country at the time.

"Hey, Catra, come over here a second," my father said.

While I wasn't quite yet a teenager, I was close and I still hated running. I hated all those soccer games. I saw my father was watching something on TV about runners. *Why does he want me to sit over there?*

"Look at these runners," he said. "These runners are running all the way from Squaw Valley all the way to Auburn."

*Whateve*r, I thought.

"Cool, Dad," I said, without much enthusiasm.

As I sat watching those runners, I thought they looked like a bunch of geeks and nerds in their short-shorts and their glasses; many of them looked sick and exhausted.

My father was not born an athlete. My grandparents were very wealthy and my grandfather was really strict. Dad's family only allowed him to play a handful of sports. My grandfather believed that golf and tennis were the only acceptable games. My grandfather never seemed happy with him. Dad went into the Army and my grandfather didn't like that; my grandfather loved golf, and Dad didn't; my grandfather didn't like the fact that Dad met my mother, a short Italian woman with a dozen brothers and sisters, and married her. He thought she was poor and he wanted Dad to marry someone in the upper crust. Dad made it his mission to act the opposite of his father. He was a super nice guy.

Later, as my brother got into soccer, my father decided he wanted to be serious about it for his son's sake and he decided to transform himself into an athlete. It was another way for him to be different than his father.

Dad read everything he could about soccer. A few years later, my father knew so much by that time that he wrote a handbook on how to coach boys' soccer.

And in order to coach soccer, Dad had to play soccer, and to play soccer, he ran.

My dad would run 5Ks, 10Ks, and half marathons regularly. He used to take my brother out with him. They used to run up Mission Peak a lot, a small but popular mountain that loomed over our town. My brother was young, but he would do these half marathons with my father.

I didn't want any part of it.

When I was going into the seventh grade, we moved to a new neighborhood and I had no friends. On the first day of attending my new school, I was standing at the bus stop, alone, like I usually was, and the other girls started talking to me. They became my new friends.

They were wild kids and they all had a lot of money, but they had sisters who were older, so that was pretty cool. We would all hang out together.

I started really getting into trouble when I was thirteen, and I was caught shoplifting. It grew from there. My dad just talked to me about it. My mother wanted to kill me.

A year later, I started smoking. I was too young to get into the nightclubs yet, so my friends and I would go to the roller-skating rink and smoke in the smoking room. I started drinking around that time and discovered boys, too. My two older sisters would buy us all alcohol.

In time, I learned how to sneak into nightclubs by lying about my age. I said I was sixteen, but I didn't look sixteen at all. I was small and skinny, but bouncers would let me in because my friends looked older.

Because of my behavior, I was growing apart from my father, but he was still always nice. He would drive me to those nightclubs sometimes, even when my mother wouldn't allow us to go.

I didn't want anything to do with my parents by the time. My dad was really goofy, and he would embarrass me if I was talking to a boy. He would come over and talk to the boy, and I hated that. But Dad was cool about it. I think he saw that teenagers have to go through certain things, and that it's usually fine, as long as they weren't out of control. Plus my parents were busy with Peggy and her drug problems.

But it got worse, I was getting in trouble for cutting school. I was really into the party scene, and I was really into myself. I would pick an outfit in a department store, and I had a friend who would steal it for me. She was so good at it, I wouldn't even see her stealing it. This went on for a while.

When I was seventeen, I wanted some money from my dad so I could buy a new outfit. My dad said no, but if I did some chores, he would give me some money. I wanted nothing to do with chores. So then he said if I brought my grades up, he would start giving me an allowance again. I got mad, said I hated him, and went to my room.

And those were the last word I said to my father.

I remember Dad getting up for work. I got off to school and went shopping afterward. I did have some money for shopping after all. I needed to pick up some shoes that I had on layaway. It was a day like any other day.

Then I got a call from Patty that Dad was in the hospital. I wasn't concerned. A month ago, he went to the hospital for the same kind of chest pain, and the doctors told him he probably had some kind of acid reflux disease, which is manageable enough.

When I got home, I got a call from my mother. My father was dead.

I got to the hospital and all I remember was being in shock. I was young still and I'd never known anyone even remotely close to me who had died. Death was something that happened to other people. I saw his body, but he didn't look dead. He looked asleep.

My mother was crying and my aunt was trying to comfort my mother, but I didn't know what to do. I just sort of stood there frozen.

My brother was completely numb, staring blankly at the floor.

As I found out later, Dad had had some chest pain and the doctor told him to go to the hospital. My boyfriend at the time had his driver's license and drove my Dad and my brother to the hospital.

A mile from the house, my father went into cardiac arrest. He was convulsing and couldn't breathe. My brother tried to help and pounded on his chest. It didn't work.

The day of the funeral, I couldn't believe how many people showed up. The church was standing room only. A few people gave eulogies and spoke so highly of him, about what a good person he was and what an inspiration he was.

I learned a lot about him that day, parts of my father that I hadn't seen before.

My brother's soccer team put a signed soccer ball in his coffin. I thought that was beautiful.

We all grieved. My mother was lost and had to start working again. My brother, who had to see Dad die in front of him, was especially quiet.

I didn't know what to do with my life without Dad's quiet direction. My mother was in a daze and busy working.

I was still only seventeen, just months after my father died, when my best friend got kicked out of high school. I chose to go to an alternative school with her. The school didn't work out, and I decided to quit and go to cosmetology school. That turned out to be a good decision in a way. I could do hair, and it was a good job. But it also allowed me to do drugs and work.

But it would take me many years before I began to love running. I would need to work at the hair salon and become a drug addict and get arrested and get better. I would search for something in my life to help me leave the drugs behind. And I would find running.

Throughout my life, I would think about this scene often. It was a fond memory of my father trying to find a way to connect with me through those awkward years when I was a bratty teenager. It's why I think Dad would have been one of those old guys running, maybe even someone in the races with me. It's also, I believe, the thing that helped lead me to run. I was looking for something to help me stay off drugs, and even many years, it's as if my father was still there, offering unwanted advice and whispering to me to help me find something that I really needed.

Chapter Four

My First Steps

In 1996, two years after I got clean and sober, I was doing well. I was working at a bagel shop, was exercising, and was going to school to get my diploma. Plus, I had a home, even if I was still living with my mother.

But I didn't have any friends. I was wrapped up in my recovery and high school and exercising to purge all those nasty, gross drugs from my system. My only companions were Oskar, my miniature dachshund, Kevin, my workout buddy who later became my boyfriend, and my mother.

The old addict me, or even the bratty teenager me, would have laughed at that. But I was a different person now. I was no longer a Goth or a clubber or much of a dancer. I was an assistant manager at a bagel shop and a high school student in her early thirties and someone who lived with her mother. It was the opposite of my old life. That, in many ways, was a good thing. So I decided to embrace this new person I'd become.

I'd been exercising for a couple years by then, lifting weights and walking Oskar three miles a day. One day, I decided I was bored with walking.

I got the idea from people running on the treadmill at the gym. That didn't look fun to me. It looked horrible actually. But I thought that maybe instead of walking those three miles with Oskar, I could try running them. There was no reason for it. I like to think it was my father whispering to me.

So the next day, I got up and put on my gym clothes. I didn't have any fancy running clothes. I had on cross-training shoes. I had no Garmin, no water bottle, no Oskar, and no idea what I was doing. But I stepped out the door and started jogging.

I felt, right away, like I was doing something. My chest felt tight. I was breathing hard. I was getting my heart rate up. This is what I wanted, so I kept going.

I didn't know anything about how to run a proper pace. I was running faster than I probably should have at the time.

When you train, you're supposed to begin running at a pace that allows you to talk. I didn't know that. I just ran.

I ran around the block, feeling as if I wanted to die.

By the time I was done, I felt overheated and exhausted. I plopped down on the front steps and took another deep breath.

I felt good.

Wow, I thought. *I ran the entire way, without walking, or stopping, or any breaks at all. I ran. I ran. I actually ran.*

I felt so good, I decided right then that I would become a runner. I wanted to be just like those people on TV who ran those big races.

Next to the bagel shop where I worked was a Barnes & Noble bookstore. On my break, I would go over there and browse through books. When you walked inside, there was a flyer board with all the different things going on in Fremont. And there was an area where you could see upcoming races, such as a bunch of 5Ks and 10Ks.

I saw on the poster board one day that there was a race called the Carousel-to-Carousel at the theme park California's Great America. I took one of the flyers and the entry form, and that night, I told my mother that I wanted to sign up for the race. I told her that she should register for the 5K walk and that I would race the 10K.

Two weeks after that first gasping run around the block, I was ready to run my first race. I didn't care that a 10K was twice as far as I'd ever run in my life. I didn't care that that first run was tough. I thought I could do it. How hard could it be?

On race day, I had some real running shoes by this point—some Reeboks I bought at a Ross clothing store—but I didn't have any other running gear. I wore my cut-off shorts and I had a black T-shirt that I usually wore when running. This was in March, but it was another hot day in California. The black T-shirt soaked in the sun. Sweat was already dripping off my nose.

I was standing at the starting line, and I looked around, and I saw all these people who looked really fit.

OK, I thought. *Well, here we go.*

At the pistol that started the race, off I went and shot off like a rocket. I still didn't know anything about how to pace myself.

I didn't stop at the water stations because I didn't know you were supposed to drink water.

I just ran as fast as I could. I just wanted to pass anyone who was next to me. I felt like I was going to die.

I finished in just over fifty minutes. I finished feeling like I was going to have a heart attack. I just collapsed on the ground right after the finish line. Someone asked if I was OK, and surprisingly, I said yes.

I felt good.

I felt great, actually.

Wow, I thought. *WOW.*

I just ran a 10K. I just ran more than six miles.

I saw my mother at the end and she was full of excitement for me.

I felt like a conquering hero.

After she congratulated me, we went to the amusement park, because you got a free ticket for running.

Another runner passed by me, and recognized me from the race.

"Why are you wearing all black?" she said.

I didn't have anything else to wear, but I didn't answer her because I was too embarrassed. I looked like a newbie, someone who obviously didn't know what she was doing. But I would change that. I would learn how to do it. I would run more. I loved the race. I wanted to do more.

We rode a couple rides in the park, but it wasn't long before I was too exhausted to continue. I just wanted to go home and crash.

As we approached my car, I saw a flier on it. I took it off, and it said SAN FRANCISCO MARATHON in big, bold letters. There was a registration form for it.

Right away, I thought of my father, who was training for his first marathon when he passed away. Seeing that registration form inspired me. *I'm going to run a marathon.*

Even though after this first 10K I thought I was going to have a heart attack and collapse and die, I also felt fantastic. I wanted that feeling again. So why not train for a race that was four times as long as the 10K?

I told my mother that I was going to run the marathon, and she just kind of looked me and said, "How far is that?"

"Oh, I don't know," I said. "About twenty miles."

"Oh my God. You're crazy," my mother said, shaking her head.

I called up Kevin, my workout buddy who was not yet my boyfriend that night, and I asked him how far a marathon actually was. He said it was 26.2 miles.

Oh man.

"Well, guess what," I said. "I'm going to sign up."

That night I clipped the registration form off the flyer that I found on my car for the San Francisco Marathon and sent in my registration check. No turning back now.

The day after I sent in my entry form, I went to my local Barnes & Noble and looked for a book on how to train for your first marathon. I grabbed the first one I saw. Mostly what I needed was a training plan. I bought the book and flipped through the pages. *Bingo!* There was a plan.

According to the training guide, runs during the weekdays of marathon training do not matter nearly as much as the runs on the weekend. (This is also true, for the most part, about ultramarathons, although I didn't know that yet.) The plans called the big weekend run a long run; that's when you really practiced for the marathon. The idea was to ease into running twenty-six miles by increasing the length of the long run every week.

My marathon was in three months. To keep on track, I needed to run nine miles on Sunday.

Oh man. The farthest I'd run, ever, was that 10K, or 6.2 miles. Now I was going to have to run three miles, or another 5K, essentially, on top of that.

It was Friday.

Back then, I didn't have anything like a GPS watch to tell me my distance. So I got in my car, set my odometer to zero, drove out until it reached 4.5 miles—halfway—and saw there was a gas station on the corner. *Perfect*, I thought. *I'll turn around at the gas station.*

That Sunday morning I put on my cut-off sweats and a cotton T-shirt, put my hair in a ponytail, and took off. When I reached the gas station, I turned around and then went back home.

When I got home, I sat down on the steps and lay down. I thought, *Wow. I just ran nine miles. Wow. I feel really good. That's what they must be talking about when they talk about a runner's high.*

I felt like a superhero.

Soon after, I decided to run another 10K on a whim and picked a trail race. It was my first trail race and only my second race ever. During the race, because I knew nothing about pacing myself, I ran really fast from the start.

About halfway through the race, with the first 5K at our backs, there was a young girl on my heels, and some old guy was yelling at her to push. He was screaming, and when she passed me, he was yelling at her not to let me catch her. Then the girl started throwing up, and the guy just kept yelling at her. *What an ass.*

She finished less than a minute ahead of me.

When I finished, I felt like my heart was going to pound out of my chest, since it was slamming through my ears. That old guy came up to me.

"Man, I thought you were going to catch us," he said. "That girl is one of our top high school runners. I'm her coach. I really had to push her. You're fast. Who are you?"

Even though I felt like I was going to die, that made me feel good. It made me feel like a runner. And not just a runner, but a pretty good one too.

His comment hit home. I was a different person now, one that I'd never thought I'd be just a couple years ago. I was a clean and sober person. I was an athlete. I was a runner. I was more like my dad than I thought.

I still didn't have any friends. So whenever someone stopped in the bagel store where I worked, and they looked like a runner, I would ask them about running.

Those runners told me about a good place to run, a nearby paved trail that wound by a creek. Plus, there were mile markers along the trail, so I could tell exactly how far I needed to go. I didn't have to drive just to mark distance anymore. It was pretty sweet.

Over the next couple of weeks, my training went well, and pretty soon, the magical twenty-mile run was on my schedule.

In most training plans, twenty miles is the farthest distance. The theory behind this is that if you can run twenty miles, then you can run a marathon.

I got up that Sunday morning, and I didn't eat or drink anything before. I ran until I got to ten miles on the trail, and then turned around.

I felt like absolute shit by the end of the run. Because of all the training I was doing, I was getting thinner and thinner. I just wasn't getting enough energy.

Two days before the San Francisco Marathon, I went to pick up my packet. My mother went with me. She was excited because we got all these free samples. One was a gel, the only one at the race expo. They were new, and I honestly didn't know what I was supposed to do with it.

"Take it at mile twenty-two," a guy told me, "when you hit the wall."

I kept hearing about this wall thing, but I didn't know what it was. When I asked, one of the race officials told me that it was the time when you would want to quit and you couldn't move.

Oh man. The wall sounded terrible.

I bought a couple new shorts at the expo. They were these new, colorful shorts, bright pink, and I got a purple shirt. I was a new person, so I needed a new look. No more black.

I was no longer a Goth dancer who did drugs to make myself feel good. I was a runner.

The day before the marathon, I was adamant about staying off my feet and keeping my legs elevated. My mom thought it was ridiculous. I drank a ton of water. That night, I had my mother cook me some mashed potatoes for some carbs.

The morning of the race, I went to the start at Golden Gate Bridge. The race course ran through all these different landmarks in San Francisco. I began to see people I recognized from other races. A woman came up to me while I was standing in line. I told her this was my first marathon.

"This is my seventy-fifth," she said and smiled. *Wow.*

I couldn't believe it. *How could anyone do that many races*, I thought.

I shivered in my singlet and shorts. Another runner offered me an extra garbage bag, which I gratefully accepted, and slipped it on and waited for the last minute, when I would take it off again and start running twenty-six miles.

And though I didn't hear the start, the runners just started moving, and so off we went.

My father often talked about the Alameda Creek Trail as he was training for his races. He loved it. I thought about him as I began to clip off the miles that would take me to the end. That was the same trail I was running now.

Halfway through the marathon, I was still feeling good and thought, *Wow, I'm becoming a marathoner.*

I'm becoming something my dad wanted to be. I was becoming one of those geeky people on TV my dad raved about, but they didn't seem so weird now. They seemed normal to me. I was becoming one of them, after all, and that made me feel closer to my father, even way after he was gone. It also made me wish he was still around so I could share it with him.

As mile twenty approached, the point where I was supposed to run into this dreaded wall, I started running by several of the nightclubs I used to go to when I was on drugs.

Back then, I had been living in a haze. The drugs were fun, and they felt good, but one of the reasons I felt euphoric all the time was because I was in a cloud that protected me from life's drudgery. The problem was that cloud concealed many other things, many wonderful things. It prevented me from seeing life's beauty. I didn't notice the hills, the mountains, or structures like the Golden Gate Bridge. I didn't notice any of the beauty that San Francisco has to offer.

Of course, there other consequences. I could have gone to jail for a long time. I could have wound up like Jason, strung out with holes in his arms, possibly dead. I could have wound up like Peggy, who lost any semblance of a normal life because of drugs. Even though I got off easy, I still lost a lot. I lost time with my family, and my mother, who I loved dearly again, and my car and many of my things and years of my life, all to the haze.

Whenever I ran by one of the clubs where I used to hang out, I'd get a new surge of energy. I remembered being in this haze and hanging with my friends and dancing.

I felt much different now as I passed by club after club. Now my euphoria was coming from my own effort. Probably for the first time in my life, I felt elation from something other than drugs.

At mile twenty-four in the marathon, the wall did come a little bit. My legs felt numb, even dead. But as I was passing by all those clubs, I kept thinking about where I was then and what I was doing now. I thought about my friends and I couldn't believe that I was still off drugs. I hoped they were all off drugs too.

A few tears ran down my face. That made me appreciate the moment as I ran. I was grateful for being able to come from this really dark place and be at the place I was at now, in this marathon with thousands of people, accomplishing something that my father would have loved to do.

Running would be a way to connect with my father, to regain the connection I lost years ago. I could no longer be daddy's little girl, but I could look back on him and appreciate what he did for me.

My legs felt heavy, even numb, but I could see the finish line. I knew my mother was waiting for me and I knew my father wouldn't be disappointed in me.

He would be so proud of me.

Once my father died, I really became a big-time partier. I was trying to numb the pain of losing a parent. My friends didn't know what to say to me. What do you say, after all, to a friend when she loses her father?

The last thing I said to my father was that I hated him. As I got older, I knew that he understood that I didn't hate him, but I was a teenager at the time and that comment fucked me up big time.

I was drinking a lot and continued to drink more and more, which is what led me to try drugs.

I thought about all this as I entered the stadium. I crossed the finish line, and I was sobbing. I couldn't believe I did it.

Thank you, Dad.

Running had become my friend. It was helping me through things. It was there for me at a time in my life when I really didn't have anything. But as I was running, I had my father by my side, helping me build this new life I had created, one without drugs. He would become my inner coach. I thought of him as my angel, guiding me, calling me peanut and telling me to go as hard as I could.

The more I ran, the more I felt connected to him. And I knew that he would probably be running right alongside me if he were still alive.

I didn't know what an ultramarathon was until I started doing it myself. I always could appreciate that my father first showed me what an ultramarathoner was that day on the couch.

But I was not yet an ultrarunner. I would have a long way to go before that. I would need to learn how to run on trails and then run trail marathons. I would face two serious health scares.

But I was a runner.

And now I was a marathoner.

Chapter Five

Disappearing One Bite at a Time

I was nine when I made my first life-altering decision.

My father always tried to make money in one way or another. My sister and I were members of 4H, and inspired by the rugged skills that we learned, he came up with a plan to buy nine steers at an auction. His plan was to fatten them up and sell them back.

My favorite one was white, like the clouds that dotted the sky above our house. I was afraid of the others, but there was something about his color that calmed me. I felt safe around him because he was super friendly. He loved to come up to me and let me pet him and touch him. I would give him hugs. I named him Charlie. We had him nearly a year. He was the last steer we kept.

One day I came home from school, my brother led me to a meat freezer that we kept in the garage.

"Hey, look in the freezer," he said.

I saw that it was full.

"What?" I said.

"Charlie's in the freezer," he said.

I was devastated.

After that, I didn't want to eat any meat my parents served me because it most likely would be Charlie. I didn't want to eat my pet. Charlie was gentle and sweet, so eating him seemed to be the opposite of that. It was a brutal act against such a kind animal.

I wasn't going to eat that animal. I didn't want to eat any animals. My mother, the great cook, would have to start worrying about her daughter's picky diet.

It would not be the last time she had to worry about it.

My two elder sisters were really pretty. So I loved being pretty and glamorous and sexy, even at a young age. I wanted to be like them.

I was just the young girl. I wanted to be older. When I was growing up in the 1970s, much like today, most actresses were thin and models were even thinner. That was how you were supposed to be glamorous and sexy. I loved the clothes they wore, so the message seemed to be that if you wanted to wear what they were wearing, you had to look like they looked. You had to look as if you were starving.

It was pretty black-and-white back then. There were no plus-size models like there are now. If you were thin, you were cute, and if you weren't, from what I could see, you were ugly.

So one day in junior high school a friend of mine brought some chocolate things that would suppress your appetite. I took them because I didn't know chocolate could do that, and I liked chocolate. But I also did it because I wanted to look like those models.

I was not a fat kid at all. But thin was in, and though it is an easy answer to blame society for that message, that is indeed what started my eating disorder. I know that a lot of young girls struggle with the way they look and diet as a result and they don't slip into an eating disorder. But the girls I hung out with were obsessed with being thin. That obsession would stick with me. It was put in my head that I had to look a certain way. It would take me many years to recover from that idea.

Once I started dating, things got even worse. My first serious boyfriend, Jim, and I were drunk all the time when we were together. We were nineteen and would go to clubs and drink every weekend. When we got home, we'd get into these big, blowout fights. We would break up and get back together every night. It was abusive, but at the time, we thought it was very romantic.

During these fights, Jim would put me down. He would call me fat, saying that I looked terrible. I quickly moved on to laxatives to lose weight.

Jim and I broke up eventually, but his words stayed with me. And I found a new way to lose weight. I started getting high. Meth was a great resource for losing weight because of the way it jacked up my metabolism.

When I moved in with Jason, I found a scale in the house. I'd never had a scale before. I became obsessed with it. It was a horrible thing for me to discover. The scale as much as anything contributed to my disorder.

I weighed as much as 120 pounds before I took drugs, but by the time we moved into his parents' house, I was down to 110. The drugs were already starting to feed my disorder. I didn't have to try to be skinny. Your metabolism gets sped up—that's why they call meth "speed"—and when I became an addict, I'd stay up for two or three days straight, dancing and working and moving around like an electron, always bouncing around, wired and buzzed. I rarely ate when I was on a binge. The pounds just dropped off. I didn't even have to try.

When I discovered the scale, I began trading weights with a friend. When she got to 109, I'd have to get to 108. I wouldn't eat for a couple days straight, and I'd get to 107, and I'd be super stoked.

When I first dropped to under one hundred pounds, I actually cheered. I had no idea that it was starting to kill me.

I stopped having periods. I would occasionally see stars when I'd stand up after sitting for a bit. My bones protruded from my skin. By the time I was arrested, I weighed only ninety-three pounds.

I stopped doing drugs after I was arrested, but I didn't have any of the mental tools to be healthy. Hell, I had no idea how to eat. And I wasn't expecting the crushing depression that came with quitting drugs and changing my lifestyle. I ate when I was sad, and some days, I didn't want to move. With no drugs, no diet plan, and no desire, I began to gain weight.

After my suicide attempt, I gained twenty pounds.

I jumped from ninety-three to 115 pounds. That sounds like a lot of weight, but 115 was a normal weight for someone my size. It was probably even a little low. But I freaked out.

I began to work out, eventually as much as three times a day. Additionally, I discovered I had a soy and wheat intolerance, which solved some stomach issues and helped motivate me to eat like a vegan. I noticed the difference. I started feeling good. The weight came off naturally because of the lifestyle changes I made. It was exactly the way you're supposed to lose weight.

But then the weight continued to drop, and I as it dropped, I ate less. I ate less, lost more weight, and I was inspired to eat even less. It was a vicious cycle.

When I began running, which quickly escalated into my first marathon, I'd feel like crap on most of my runs, especially my long runs. But I thought that's how you were supposed to feel. You were running for as long as three or four hours on those long runs. Who didn't feel like crap while you running that long?

As I began running more, the weight dropped off even faster. I ate a few pieces of fruit a day, and then I cut down to three apples a day.

The positive feedback I got made things worse at first. Kevin, my workout partner and later my boyfriend, was a good guy. He supported me and was nice to me. But that support only fed my eating disorder more. He complimented me the skinnier I got.

"You look great, babe," he would tell me as the pounds came off. I wouldn't eat, and I'd hear something nice from Kevin, and then I would run these races, and I would feel good about myself.

Just like Jim, he helped feed my eating disorder. Kindly intentioned words can damage someone just as much as mean ones.

At the end of my first marathon, I was down to ninety-seven pounds.

I began using laxatives to keep my weight below a hundred pounds.

People began to notice as my bones once again poked my skin. They would say that I looked sick. I developed an excuse, and it became my go-to answer whenever someone would say something about my weight.

I was a vegan and a runner.

I'd go to parties for work all the time, and people would offer food, and I'd turn them down, explaining that I was a vegan. When they said that I looked thin and hungry, I'd explain that I was a runner. Runners just look that way.

I stopped having periods again, and my doctor warned me about my weight during one of my appointments. She asked if I have an eating disorder.

No, I'd answer. I was a vegan and I ran.

My therapist looked me over one day and asked if I had a disorder.

No, I answered, I'm a vegan and I run.

Pretty soon, it became the excuse I would use for myself as well. I didn't have to worry about feeling like crap on my long runs, even as I began training for ultramarathons. I was a vegan and a runner. I didn't have to worry about my body rebelling. I was a vegan and a runner.

I didn't have to worry about what others thought. I didn't have to worry about those nagging thoughts in the back of my head that this was now an addiction and that, if I didn't seek help for it, I could die.

I was a vegan and a runner. But I was also a woman in the throes of another kind of addiction. It would take time, treatment, and the same kind of will power I had to demonstrate to finish my ultramarathons to get better.

Chapter Six

Back to School

When I was sitting at the table with my mother, enduring her wrath, listening to her telling me how upset she was with me for doing drugs, she said one thing to intentionally hurt me.

"Your father would be very disappointed in you," she seethed through her teeth.

I knew my addiction would be disappointing, which is why I didn't want to tell her. It's also why I only saw her once a month, too. I didn't want her to figure out that I was on drugs.

But I needed to stay at her place, a safe place, for my recovery. I needed to get away from Jason and away from my friends who wanted me to do drugs. I needed some support, as I had just tried to kill myself.

I needed her.

I was a daddy's girl growing up and that's because it always seemed Dad let me do what I wanted. He said yes a lot.

But my mother had a harder edge. She was quick to say no, so we clashed a lot.

When I was little, if I fell and scraped my knee, I would start crying. I was sensitive and soft. My mother seemed to be the opposite.

My mother had to be tough. She was the youngest of a dozen kids. She had to learn how to scrap, and she bonded the most with a brother who was a couple years older than her and loved sports. She played basketball and field hockey. She was used to bruises.

When I scraped my knee, she would tell me I was fine. It was just a scrape. "Suck it up," she would tell me. But I didn't want to hear that. I wanted someone to coddle me.

Later, when I started dating, she would hound me to stick up for myself. She would nag me to do what I wanted to do, not just what my guy wanted to do. But I wasn't like that. I would do what he wanted. She hated that.

"You have a voice," she would tell me. "You can say no."

But my mother was also sweet in her own way. The kids in my neighborhood loved her because she would always make anyone food. She loved cooking and was good at it.

She was a hard-edged and tough but loving and positive person. And when I needed to recover, that's exactly what I needed in my life. I rejected a lot of her mothering when I was a teen, but I needed it now.

I understood why she was chewing me out. It was hard to hear, but I loved to hear it as well.

The good news, I told her, was that I was off the drugs, and I was going to rebuild my life.

My mother was supportive but skeptical. She had heard all this before from Peggy.

In order to rebuild my relationship with my mother, I would need to prove myself to her. I would need to stay clean and sober. I would need to continue to run and work hard at my job, at life, and show her the new person I'd become.

And the first step to all that was going back to school.

On my first day of going back to high school, my mother asked me a question. "Why don't you just go back and get your GED?"

That's what most adults do, after all. But I didn't want to do it that way. I actually wanted to get my high school diploma.

I was about to head back to class, where I would enter my old elementary school and work hard at my studies for the first time in my life. I was going to do what I should have done back when I was a teenager. That's what I needed to do. It was the first step to getting my life back. In some ways, it was the only way to build a new life, the one I should have lived twenty years ago.

The school itself, in many ways, still looked like the school I attended when I was a little girl. There were still murals on the walls and the short little water fountains, and it had that same musty, old smell.

I walked in and sat in the front row.

I was finally ready to listen.

The teachers I had for my GED were amazing. I told them my story when they would ask, but it wasn't just about bragging about how far I'd come. I needed them to hold me accountable to staying clean and sober and as free from depression as I could manage. Drugs lurked. Depression lurked. Desire lurked.

I felt as if I had some good teachers for the first time in my life, who really cared about me and wanted me to do well. They wanted me to succeed.

Even so, it was a little bit scary. I was an adult, and I was going to school with kids who had been kicked out of school, rough hooligans who would stare me down when I passed them in hallway. There were some sad cases. One girl with some sort of mental illness would come in with makeup smeared on her face and would talk to herself and have outbursts. At first I thought she was doing it on purpose, but later, I figured out that she couldn't help it, and I began to feel sorry for her.

There were also a lot of immigrants, people from India, China, and Vietnam who were trying to learn English.

Going to school during the day kept me on track. I needed to get up in the morning and run and go to school and then go to the bagel shop where I worked. I needed the routine to stay clean and make my mother proud.

I went for two years, and I was able to graduate, and one day, the principal called for me to go to the office. She asked me if I would be the valedictorian.

I was friggin' thrilled.

Growing up, even if I had been much more motivated, there was no way I would have been able to be a valedictorian. I wasn't that smart, and I wasn't motivated. Not only did I not want to work hard, I didn't want to work at all.

But my teachers voted for me to be the valedictorian. They didn't have many cases like me, people who were older and wanted to make a new life and were successful at it.

I started crying. I felt so honored.

Then they told me I needed to prepare a speech.

Gulp.

But immediately, I knew what I would talk about.

I would talk about my life.

At graduation, I stood up and took a deep breath before my speech, and then I talked about what I'd been through. I talked about the drugs I'd taken and my father, and how I wanted to become someone I deserved to be. My teachers all hugged me after I was finished talking. One student came up to me after and said my story inspired her. She was battling drugs, too, she said, and it helped to hear from someone who had truly beaten them. My mother, however, was embarrassed. She looked at my drug problem as a glitch in my life. She didn't understand why I would want to talk about such a flaw.

Because I was valedictorian, the school paid for a semester of college. My first day, I walked through the front door and prepared to be a physical therapist. I sat in the front row. I was ready to listen.

And I stared out the window and looked at the trail up to Mission Peak.

It was so hard for me to concentrate. The motivation for working hard in class was gone. I had proven to myself and to my mother, at least partly. I no longer needed the routine. I didn't want to be a physical therapist.

I wanted to be outside, on Mission Peak, on the trail.

I had a different calling.

Chapter Seven

Molested

No one wants to be a drug addict.

At least, I don't think anyone does. Granted, the lifestyle was fun for me. The partying was fun. The nightclubs were fun. The buzz in my head, and the good feelings that seeped from it, were all fun. The friends I had because of drugs were fun. But the drugs? Not fun. They damaged my relationship with my mother, destroyed the relationship we had with my sister and probably would have ended my life had I not gotten thrown in jail and not became an ultrarunner. Those moments were when I figured out that I didn't want to be a drug addict. And that's when I also figured out that I never really did enjoy being a drug addict. Some addicts, like my sister, unfortunately never figure that out. Others figure it out too late. I was lucky. I figured it out in time to rebuild my life. I became a new person.

While no one wants to become a drug addict, years later my therapist told me why people tend to become one. They become addicts, she said, because something is wrong. It's either something that is going on in their lives, or it's something that happened in their past. They use drugs to help them forget about those problems.

At least, that's why I used drugs, my therapist said. The drugs were fun, but they were mostly a tool.

They helped me forget about something horrible that happened to me when I was a little girl.

My oldest sister, Patty, was getting married in 1972. I was nine, and because I was only nine, I was a little sad I wasn't in the wedding party.

Peggy and Jay were both in it, but I was at an in-between age. I was too old to be a flower girl and too young for anything else.

But I did get to wear a really cute dress. It was long and peach-colored, and I got to wear my black, shiny shoes. My hope was that my sister would have a baby, because that's what people did when they got married, and then I would have a little sister. It wasn't all bad.

In fact, the wedding was amazing, and the reception back at our house was awesome. Everyone was having fun and dancing, and so was I, in my black, shiny shoes. Everyone had a lot of fun.

One guest at the wedding was Steve, a family friend. I knew him well since he was around the house a lot, doing odd jobs. He was nice, friendly, and funny.

But he also drank a lot, mostly Coors.

That night, after the wedding, Steve was drinking a lot more usual, and more than just Coors. He was drunk, like he seemed to be a lot. He passed out on the couch, and my parents eventually went to bed.

While I was sleeping that night, my door opened, and the squeak of the hinges woke me up, and I heard someone come into my room. It was dark, and I couldn't see who it was, but I could feel someone over me. Then he started talking to me. I could tell it was a man because of his low voice. And then I smelled the Coors on his breath.

Steve's voice.

Steve's hands slipped under my covers, and he started touching me. He began rubbing my vagina, and his beer breath washed over my small face, telling me not to say anything. I didn't say anything. I pretended I was asleep. I didn't know what else to do. I was frozen in fear.

I tried to pretend that Steve wasn't there and touching me and making me feel horribly uncomfortable. I'd never before had any reasons to be really, really scared. I had no idea why he was touching me that way, and why he was telling me, in his low voice, that I couldn't tell anyone about it because something really bad would happen to my family.

I didn't want anything bad to happen to my family. So I just lay there and tried to be as quiet as I could. It was my only defense.

Steve got up, and I hoped he would leave. *Please leave*, I thought, trying not to cry. *Please just leave.* He got up and stumbled a bit to my closet, and he started peeing in there. I wrinkled my noise against the mix of vinegar and sweat and Coors. He leaned by my side and started touching me again.

He was in there about fifteen minutes and I could see a light go on through my partially opened door. When he was done, he got up and scurried out of my bedroom, like a rat.

"What are you doing?" I heard my Dad ask.

"I was trying to find the bathroom," Steve answered.

I wanted to cry out to "Daddy," but I lay there, still and silent, and hoped he would not come back in. I somehow fell asleep.

When I woke up, the sun was sneaking in through the windows. He was gone.

A couple hours later, my mother asked me a question offhand, in between the rush of our daily life.

"Was Steve in your room last night?" she asked.

Here was my chance to tell her and let go of the weight that would crush me for years. But I was nine, and all I could think about was something happening to my family and how horrible I would feel when it happened because it would be my fault.

"No," I answered.

Nothing ever happened again with Steve, but I never wanted to be alone around him ever again. I avoided situations where I knew I might be alone around him. And I always carried the horrible memory with me. The shame and the guilt and the fact that somehow I must have caused what happened to me. I put my family in danger. I put myself in danger. I would not let that happen again.

I never said anything to anyone. I remained frozen with fear. I was silent and still, just like that night.

Steve, as it turns out, was a huge creep. First of all, he dated a lot of younger girls. When I was in high school, he was dating a girl who went to my high school. He remained a friend of the family and would even buy alcohol for us at times.

A few years later, he was dating a woman in our neighborhood and she caught him molesting her daughter. Many years later, after my Dad had died, he went to prison for molesting his son.

He was a complete fucking pervert, apparently, and that only added to my guilt for not saying something. Maybe if I had, that wouldn't have happened to those other kids.

But I didn't say anything, and I had to go through life with this big secret, and it fucked me up for many years. I think that's part of the reason why I began drinking and experimenting with drugs. I tried to stuff the pain inside me, and I tried to keep it stuffed down with drugs and alcohol.

I never, ever drank beer. The smell of it made me sick, probably because of Steve. It always smelled like the stink of someone stripping away the innocence of a little girl.

But that is why getting arrested was the best thing that happened to me. I got help. I got off drugs, and in order to stay off drugs, I went to a therapist.

After the therapist helped me by emphasizing obvious but true statements, like 'you can't change the past' and that it was understandable that I didn't say anything when it happened, she said I needed to tell my mother what had happened. It had bothered me throughout my life. In many ways, it led to my drug addiction. She thought I needed to move on with my life, and telling my mother, she said, would help me do that. Twenty years after I was molested, I had to tell my mother what happened to me.

I knew the conversation would be tough, but it wouldn't be as bad as telling her that I was a drug addict. At least I was clean and sober at this point.

My mother's reaction was predictable. She was angry.

"Why didn't you tell us?" she asked me.

She wasn't as mad as she was when I told her I was an addict, of course, but she was upset. But I could feel some regret there, too, as if she should have found out what had happened or even prevented it. I think she felt bad.

But telling my mother made a huge difference. It helped me to put the assault behind me. I could move on. Other people had way more traumatic experiences than me, I realized. I could move on from something like that.

Later, my mother would tell me that it helped her to know why I did drugs. Even though it made her sad, it also helped her to know that I turned to drugs partly to help me forget about what happened. She always blamed herself for Peggy, but it was nice for my mother to know that it wasn't her fault that I turned to drugs.

Throughout my life, as I went through relationships, I was always looking for someone to make me feel better about myself. I had boyfriends constantly, and it drove my mother crazy because I gave into them all the time. The relationships never seemed to be healthy. They were verbally and sometimes physically abusive. I never felt good about myself, and I was insecure.

I felt ready to have a real relationship once I told my mother about what happened.

Chapter Eight

Learning to Be Tough on the Trail

After I finished my first marathon, my mother said she was really proud of me. And then she said something that showed she didn't really understand all my running.

"Now you don't have to do another," she said.

The thing was, she was wrong. I did need to do another one, and another one after that. I needed it in ways that most people, including my mother, didn't understand.

By the time I was scheduled to run the Honolulu Marathon in 1996, I was probably the only one who understood what running was doing for me. I wanted to run as many marathons as I could because it made me feel good about myself. Completing marathons gave me the same kind of elation that the drugs gave me, except running was improving my life, not fucking it up. It made all the difference.

Even back then, before ultramarathons became popular, there were many races on the thousands of miles of trails that snaked across my state. And that's how I began to discover the trails around the city.

I began to run at this place called Coyote Hills, which had a six-mile loop around a dirt path. It wasn't really over the mountains like Mission

Peak that I climbed by following my father's ghost, but it wasn't asphalt. It was a trail and I visited regularly.

I enjoyed the trails. They were in beautiful areas that I'd never seen before. I was a city girl who hung out in clubs and discos with drug addicts. The trails were a completely different place. They were the opposite of my former life, and that fit, since I was trying to build a life that was the opposite of the dangerous one I'd led before I got arrested. I had a goal of running all the marathons held in California by this point in my life, and I knew that I would need to run some of those marathons on trails in order to achieve that goal. But I was ready for it. I was ready to take my first steps to becoming an ultramarathoner.

The morning of my first trail marathon, it was pouring, and my mother was along with me in the front seat. I couldn't see out the front windshield as the wipers tried in vain to shove aside the sheets of rain.

"There's no way they will have a race," my mother said.

We waited in the car at the start. The rain only seemed to be getting worse, like someone was pouring buckets over my car. The start time came, and then it went, and then the race director knocked on our window a few minutes later.

"The rangers won't let us run," he said. "The race is canceled."

My mother seemed satisfied with that answer, but I wasn't. I was pissed. I drove my mother home and then paced about the house with my jacket on. I was ready to run. I wanted to run.

I wasn't willing to let my first trail marathon get rained out.

"What are you going to do?" my mother asked, incredulously.

I was going to run a marathon.

"You're crazy," my mother said.

She really didn't understand.

I got dressed in my normal workout clothes and drove out to Coyote Hills, and I stepped out into the pouring rain. I came to run a marathon, and, fuck it, I was going to run a marathon.

About halfway through my run, the rain fell so hard it felt like a cold shower. With water running off my nose like a gutter, plunging through my shirt and soaking my eyelids, I realized that I was probably a little different. I didn't know then that I was destined to do what I'm doing now, but this was the first sign that I wasn't going to stop running, and that, in fact, I was just going to get crazier. I was willing to put myself through situations that most people would consider torture.

I didn't know anyone who ran yet, so I didn't have any reason to be out there other than my own internal hunger. I didn't need company to love the misery. I was truly different than I was years ago when I was a little girl who cried when I scraped my knee. I was like my mother now. I loved it. I was a lot more like my mother than I realized. I was now tough.

It made me appreciate my mother a lot more. There was a lot of her in me, and discovering that her toughness was inside me all this time made me take a look at the other parts of her life and how she influenced me. Living with her now helped me get to know her through long talks over dinner after she cooked for me.

When my mother was in high school, she and her friends loved to look glamorous like Marilyn Monroe. With hair curled down to their necks, they wore beautiful dresses that emphasized their small waists and showed just enough of their high-heeled pumps over sexy ankles.

I loved to look glamorous like her. At first, and for many years, that meant dressing like a vampire, with a face coated in white makeup and black lipstick. It meant working as a go-go dancer, in black lace and boots up to my hips. As I continued to form my new identity as a trail runner and marathoner, I finally ditched the black T-shirts. I still wanted to look pretty, but I would find a new look. I began to look for colorful shorts and tops to wear at races. I looked stylish and tough at the same time. It made me feel alive and energetic, the same way my mother felt when dressing like Monroe.

I wore something pink, instead of black, to my first official trail marathon after the one I ran on my own. My whole outfit was pink. Even my hair was pink.

My mother, as she always did, went with me to the race to show her support, even if she didn't understand the running itself.

During this race, it was sunny and warm, without a cloud in the sky. There was no chance of being rained out, so nothing would save me now. This one would be tough. The course was over mountains and hills and hard, rocky dirt trails, the kind that punished feet and lungs. It was my first experience with the kind of trails that would make me the ultrarunner I would become.

At the start, I melted into the center of a small group of runners. It was a group you could get lost in. Here was a handful of hard runners, who looked me over and smiled at me. They made me nervous.

From the start, I frantically looked from one ribbon to the next that marked the trail, trying not to get lost. I ran up rocks and over a thin, single trail no wider than my thin, bony frame, and the trail seemed to keep going as I ran it, like it was taunting me. It was like running on a treadmill of dirt and stone. It just kept going.

I saw my mother as I completed the first loop of the race.

"Oh good," my mother said. "You're done. That took a while."

But I wasn't done. I was only halfway done and told her so.

"What?" she said. "Why is this taking so long?"

Even though Mom didn't understand running, she was right in this case: I had been running for three hours. I normally finished my marathons in around four hours. This was different.

"Hey," I yelled back. "This is the hardest thing I've ever done. There are hills and all kinds of climbing and shit, Mom."

It was, indeed, the hardest thing I'd ever done at that point.

I was beat up, dusty, and hot, and my feet hurt. Running on trails was hard, and even running my first trail marathon through a heavy rainstorm didn't seem as hard as this. It was rocky and hilly and hot, and it was stressful, too, because there were no spectators or even enough runners to lead you the right away. The trail could lead you astray. It wasn't just one obvious path through a city with thousands of runners around you. I looked for the ribbons that race directors tied to bushes and frantically hoped I would see the next one. When I did, I felt a tinge of relief and then began to stress about seeing the next one.

About halfway through the second loop, sure enough, my worst fears came true. It was a long time between ribbons. Did I miss one? I missed one, I realized with a sinking heart. I began to panic. I was lost. I began to wander back on the trail, like a kid in a mall without her mother, until I heard a voice. "Catra?"

I looked up and saw the old man who reminded me of my own father.

"Jim!" I said, excitedly. It was great to see such a familiar face.

We found our way back to the course together. It was nice to have someone to run with. I needed it. I was tired and needed to talk to someone to take my mind off the pain as I slogged through the trail. When I finished, I realized two things: I needed a lot more practice on the trails, and I loved running on a trail. I wasn't sure I would run another race on the road again.

My mother hugged me at the finish. "Finally!" she said and smiled. "That seemed really hard."

Mom didn't understand my running. She even questioned it, especially as my weight slipped off me and my skin turned to bones. She would tell me all the time that I ran too much.

But she would tell all her friends about my running. She was proud of me.

I think she knew why it was good for me: it was because I was becoming the person she always wished I would become. I was no longer Catra the drug addict, or Catra the Goth. I was Catra the daughter and Catra the runner. That's who I was now. Running was now a part of my identity.

Running gave me something to focus on. Even though it became like an addiction, it was not an addiction. I didn't need to do it to avoid the pain of coming off a high. I wanted to do it. It was my choice. Unlike the drugs, it was something that made me a better person. It made me healthier and happier, and it made me feel like I could take on anything. I could even rebuild my life with my mother's help.

I loved laying out of my clothes to get ready when I would wake up at dawn, a time when I'd just be going to bed in my former life. I was organized. I had a plan. I was always training for something. I had a plan for my life. I had what I needed.

Most of all, it was a way to connect with my mother again and prove to her that I really did want to change my life. I really could become the tough, hard-working person that she'd always been.

It can take us many years before we appreciate our parents. Sometimes that means going to college and seeing a pile of laundry grow in a corner. Sometimes it means getting our first job and our first apartment and wondering how we were going to get dinner that night. For me, it took dropping out of high school, a drug habit, and a couple marathons. But now I appreciated my mother.

I began working at Whole Foods, my first job with a future, and I was ready to live on my own, but I decided to stay at home and enjoy the time that we'd never had together. I wanted to help my mom, keep her company and enjoy her positive influence. I paid her rent for my bedroom. We built a fun life together. We would going shopping or to the movies together, and we would go to the cemetery and put flowers on my father's grave.

On birthdays, I'd take her to dinner; on Halloween she would decorate the house with her cheesy, funky, scary stuff; on Christmas, we would wake up and open our presents, and she would dress up in a festive sweater.

I began to run a lot more too. And even though she didn't understand it, she saw herself in me.

After that trail marathon, after she greeted me at the finish, when I was sweaty and exhausted and limping back to the car, my mother looked me over and smiled. She knew I had dug deep.

"You get that from me," she said and smiled.

Chapter Nine

Becoming an Ultrarunner

While running that trail marathon, I overheard other runners talking about ultramarathons. When I asked them what those were, they replied ultras were races longer than a marathon. That sounded crazy to me. But it also sounded intriguing. I began to think about doing one as soon as I crossed the finish line.

A 50K is just under thirty-two miles. How much harder would an additional six miles be?

This attitude of being able to conquer any distance would help me start to do some crazy things right away. But it would also occasionally get me into trouble. As it would turn out, a 50K was way different. Races of that length are almost always on trails, and as I'd already discovered, trail marathons were way different than road marathons. When running one, you have to conserve your energy even more than during a marathon. A 50K is just six miles longer, but remember, most marathoners suffer a lot in those last six miles. Now I would be tacking on another six. I'd have to learn how to train for that and race through that agony.

First, I had to enter a race.

I called the race director of the Ohlone Wilderness 50K, one of the races I heard others mention many times, and told him I was interested in running his race. This was generally how you entered races back before the internet: there was no online registration.

He asked me how many ultras I'd done. I told him zero. I could hear him chuckle on the other end in response.

"This isn't a good one to do for your first time," he said.

Ohlone had many, many thousands of feet in elevation gain and was rocky and tough.

He recommended the Skyline 50K Endurance Run. That one was much tamer, he said, even if it was also be a challenge.

Alright then.

It was not the only thing I'd have to learn at the Skyline 50K, a race that wound through the Oakland Hills.

My training was not much different than one I did for a marathon. I did my usual twenty-mile long runs and thought that would be enough. It was enough, but I would have a lot to learn.

When the gun went off, I felt pretty good in the beginning, but as the race went on, the heat started to climb higher and faster than the hills that accompanied the course. It spiked to 100 degrees. I charged up those hills, and I passed somebody who shook his head as I stormed by.

"Is this your first 50K?" he said.

Indeed it was.

"You should be walking these hills," he told me.

I refused to listen. This was a race, not a hike, and I wasn't going to walk in a race. I was going to run those hills. I would pay for that later.

As the race went on, I wasn't drinking or eating anything and the heat made my face hot and wet and crusty with salt.

I still didn't want to eat anything because of my eating disorder. But my body began to get weaker and weaker, and finally when I got the next aid station, I choked down some bananas. My insides felt like they were baking, and I started to drink a lot of water.

Those last six miles were agony. I almost crawled to the finish. But I did finish.

I'd already made myself into a pretty accomplished runner, especially when I compared myself with 99 percent of the population. I'd run a few marathons, two of them on trails. But my inexperience showed the most in my diet, especially during the Skyline. I still had no idea how to fuel myself during the long runs required to train for a race like a marathon, and I especially had no idea to give my body the fluids and nutrients it needed to get me through that 50K.

This is harder than it seems. Just eat, right? It's not that simple. Many long-distance runners, even those without eating issues, struggle to eat during a race. The intense physical demands of a long race can make your stomach sensitive to anything. Runners get achy tummies or feel nauseous, and it's not unusual for them to vomit during a long race. As a result, runners have to learn how to eat during one. They learn by eating during their training runs and discovering what works and how much they can eat. I suffered through my training runs, without eating, because I still wasn't ready to confront my disorder.

One day, I was on a long run, training for this first 50K, during the middle of a really hot, California day. I didn't have any water with me, and I didn't bring anything to eat. All of the sudden, I felt a flutter in my chest. And then it felt like someone released a box of horseflies around my heart.

Little pink and white dots started exploding before my eyes. Some call that "seeing stars," but it was more violent than that. I stopped running and sat down and put my head between my legs.

I got up and slowly started running again. Then I ran some more and felt okay.

The episode shook me since my father died at such a young age of a heart attack.

But it didn't shake me up enough; I didn't do anything about it.

I refused to listen to my body. As I began to run ultramarathons, that would all start to catch up to me.

Not only was I catching up in the race, I was catching up from months of refusing to feed my body to overcome all the punishment I was putting through it. And yet I would continue to ignore the warning signs until I had to make a choice.

The ultrarunning series was not what it is today. Today you could find at least a 50K to run every weekend in California. Back then, in 1998, there were only a few held during the summer and into the fall. If you wanted to compete in multiple races, you had to run them all in a row, back-to-back almost. That's why I found myself entered in the Tampala Headlands 50K two weeks after the Skyline. Most everyone who liked to compete in ultras did this back then. You entered as many races as you could to take advantage of the season. There's a saying that you can rest when you're dead: in this case, you could just rest in the winter, when no races were offered. Sure enough, I felt strong enough to finish Tampala.

Competing like this is something that no one would recommend. As an ultrarunner, you usually train for one specific race, recover, and then do another one. This helps you avoid injury and burnout. I didn't know anything about that. I just knew I'd found a new interest and I wanted to be immersed in it.

Since I knew I could do a 50K, I figured I could do a fifty-miler, and so a month after my second 50K, I was ready to do the Firetrails 50, a fifty-mile race that uses generally the same course through the Oakland Hills as Skyline does. I finished it without any huge issues, and two weeks later, I decided to do another fifty-miler.

The morning of my second fifty-miler in the Napa Valley, in November 1998, my boyfriend, Kevin, watched me look at the window as a cold, crashing rain dumped outside my hotel room door. It reminded me of my first trail marathon, the one that I ran by myself after the official race was washed out. That run that led me to discover that I was different than most people, that special run where I discovered my toughness and willingness to suffer.

A hundred-miler was a magic milestone for me. I looked at that distance the same way many runners looked at the marathon: it was the ultimate goal, one that would define them as a true runner. I looked at the hundred-miler the same way: if I could do a hundred-miler, then I could call myself an ultramarathoner. I wanted to call myself that badly. In my mind, if I was an ultramarathoner, I was no longer a drug addict. I could truly leave that identity behind.

A hundred-miler seemed both impossible and within reach at the same time. It seemed impossible because it was hundred miles. It was three times as long as a 50K. And yet it also seemed within reach because

I could suffer through anything. I could run twenty-six miles through a cold shower.

I was tough, like my mom.

I would need every bit of that toughness as I looked outside the window, with the rain smashed into it, as if an ocean was crashing waves into the pavement outside.

And I made a deal with myself. If I could run a fifty-miler through this, in the cold, wet misery created by this deluge, I would sign up for a hundred. It would mean I was ready.

I took the option to run an hour before the official start, a gift to those who weren't sure if they could finish by the cutoff, but that meant I'd be starting in the dark.

As the rain slammed into the hotel windows, Kevin attempted to be the voice of reason, just like he would many times in my future races. He asked me if I was seriously about to run the race.

To be fair to Kevin, the race directors did talk about canceling the race, since it was pouring with no sign of letting up. But because this was an ultramarathon and the runners are used to suffering, the directors decided to put it on. I was happy about it because I was ready to run. Hell, I'd run in the rain before.

So I took my crappy flashlight to the start. Rain flooded my face and stole my breath whenever I looked up from the ground. I could see the storm approaching in the dark, and the light barely cut through the film of the monstrous, angry water.

The gun sent us off, into the dark, cold rain, and three steps into the race, I fell knee-deep into a puddle. Three seconds into the race, I was shivering and soaked. I got up, but soon after, it began to hail.

I didn't have the right equipment to repel the storm. All I had were road running shoes and purple shorts and a windbreaker. I bought the windbreaker at a thrift store. It was all I could afford.

Still, I gutted my way through it, and as the course wound back to the end of the 50K, I had a decision to make.

The second lap would take me out again, away from the warmth of a room and a shower and dry clothes. Many of the runners decided to give in to the conditions and stop at the 50K.

These were seasoned, hardscrabble ultrarunners who had initially decided to run the fifty miles and trained their butts off to do it. And yet, they stopped because the conditions warranted that. Many were so cold and wet and miserable that they decided to drop out. By that point, it was like running through a sea.

But conquering that distance didn't mean as much to many of them as it did to me. I was shivering, too, but I really wanted to test myself. This was a turning point in my life. I could stop and be just a runner and a former drug addict, or I could make myself into an ultrarunner and truly leave my past behind. I had a deal with myself.

So I decided to go back out and run the extra twenty miles.

I hung in there and kept running, and if I needed another sign that I made the right decision and that that moment would truly change my life, well, I got one in the last seven miles. The sun came out, the birds started chirping, and it was warm and beautiful. I finished in last place, but I did finish. When I got back to my hotel room, I was pumped. Excitedly, I flipped through an issue of *Ultrarunning* magazine and searched until I found an entry for another hundred-miler. I sent in my registration the next day.

I was not yet an ultrarunner, at least not in my mind. But I was ready to give it a shot.

But before I could, I would have to address something else.

Before I finished running that day, I passed another runner, and we started talking. I told him about my desire to run a hundred, and he looked me over.

"You're too skinny to run a hundred miles," he said.

His comment shocked me. *What? Weren't all runners skinny?*

"You've got to put on some weight," he said. "You're going to need that extra fat."

I'd considered that thought before. On a couple hot training runs over the last few months, I'd had some scary episodes.

The stress of training was bad enough, but my eating disorder had turned me into a skeleton, literally, of my former self. Even worse, I was using laxatives to control my weight and eating at most three apples a day. I was under a hundred pounds.

When you run a hundred miles, he told me, you'd be on your feet for a whole day and a whole night and probably another day after that. You might puke, and you wouldn't eat much, and you'd be moving the entire time if you wanted to finish. You'd have to have some calories in the bank in order to make it.

I thought about what he said. It stuck with me.

I thought I had passed my biggest test to becoming an ultrarunner by finishing that fifty-miler. But I was wrong.

In order to become an ultrarunner, I would need to figure out how to beat my eating disorder.

Chapter Ten

One Bite at a Time

"Carol?" my mother said to me one morning.

I knew right away that she was worried. She only called me by my birth name when she was upset.

Once again, it was my sister, Peggy, who talked to my mother about my weight.

"Catra is on drugs again," she said to my mother. But Mom knew she was wrong.

"She's just running," my mother said, putting her off.

By this time my mother mostly accepted the excuse as well. I was a vegan and a runner. There was no need to worry.

But she also couldn't help but notice the skin hanging off my bones. She couldn't help but notice that during a trip to New York, where my mother received an award for work, that I didn't eat anything during the lavish banquet. She couldn't help but notice that by the time I ran my second fifty-miler, I was down to eighty-nine pounds.

"Carol," my mother said. "I never see you eat."

And she was mostly right. Even when I did eat, it was mostly binge-ing and purging. If I did eat, I'd take a laxative later.

I didn't tell her about the episode with my heart while training for the 50K, and so of course I refused to acknowledge it when I had three more episodes like it.

And it was only getting worse. One day I decided to rollerblade to the gym. I would run on the treadmill, lift some weights, and then rollerblade home. It was 100 degrees outside. I rollerbladed home and my heart started to flutter again. When I got back to my mother's, I got super dizzy.

And then I blacked out.

When I came to, my mother was standing over me.

"What the hell is wrong with you?" she said. "Why are you rollerblading in this heat?"

I was putting my body through some gritty, almost impossible things, and I was not feeding it anything to help it recover. An apple a day does not always keep the doctor away, especially if that's all you're eating a day; many times that's all I was eating.

I was terrified to hear what the doctor would say about my heart, but I knew I had to go. I didn't want to wind up like my father. I was in my mid-thirties and wasn't that much younger than he was when he died. That fact was all I thought about before my second fifty-miler. I was afraid to eat because I didn't want to gain weight, and I was afraid I had to start eating because I didn't want to die of a heart attack like my father did.

My fears boxed one another, in round after round, slugging into a stalemate, until that runner and I began talking in the pouring rain during that second fifty-miler.

"You're too skinny," the man said. "There's no way you'll be able to do a hundred-miler."

That was the kick in the ass that I needed.

I knew that in order to beat my eating disorder, I would need to treat it like an addiction. It was an addiction. It fit every definition of the word. I was doing something despite the harm it was causing me.

By this point, I hadn't had a period in years. My hair was falling out. I was eighty-three pounds.

I read up on anorexia, and it was scary to see what could happen to me. I could die. I wasn't that far from it, from what I could read. I definitely wouldn't be able to train and complete a hundred-miler without beating it.

I realized I needed help. The first step, of course, with any addiction is admitting that you have a problem. I bought a book on nutrition. I began to eat a little bit more here and there. It helped to approach it like my training. When I went for a long run, I would eat as many calories as I would need to cover what I would burn on the long run. It wasn't eating so much as it was training.

Food is fine, I told myself. *You need fuel.*

I continued to read about what to eat. It was amazing how little I knew about eating right and appropriately fueling my body for an ultra-marathon. By this point I'd run many marathons and two fifty-milers, and yet, I didn't know much about how you needed carbs to fuel your body and protein to help it recover.

I looked into supplements, which is what led me to Whole Foods and a career with the store. I didn't give up my vegan diet, but I learned about food like almond butter, items that had the fat and calories I needed. I began to eat it by the spoonful.

It did help that this was just the way I was. I just asked myself if I wanted to live or die. I didn't want to die. It was the same approach that got me off drugs. I didn't want to spend another night in jail, so I gave them up.

But it was not that easy, and I knew it. I began working the other steps to a twelve-step program. That was the only way I knew to beat an addiction. I had to admit that I couldn't control it, and I looked back on my past. I made amends with people and apologized to many of them, including my mother, for lying about my condition and telling them I was just a vegan and a runner when I was actually an addict.

I struggled, and in some ways, I struggled more with this addiction than my addiction to drugs. It was hard when I started to put on weight. It felt weird. It felt wrong in some ways.

I'd still step on the scale every morning, and it was very hard to see the numbers go up, even though that meant that I was in recovery. It was what my body needed, but the scale was powerful. It continued to haunt me. When I'd gain a couple pounds, it made me depressed, not happy. I was anxious about it, like I was doing something wrong.

I was weighing myself every day.

Even when people tried to be supportive, such as my mother, it would mess with my head.

"You're gaining weight!" she said to me a few weeks into my recovery.

I took that as I was getting fat.

But I did notice something important. During my long runs—at this point, they would last all day, up to forty miles or more—I would feel good. I began to have more energy during the week too. I no longer felt like crap. It made the runs a lot more fun. I even began to really enjoy them. It made the hundred-miler seem possible.

So I knew the program was working. And so I knew what I would have to do.

I would have to get rid of my tangible nemesis.

One morning, I walked into the bathroom and grabbed the scale.

The scale continued to eat at me. It tried to control me every day. When I would see it, I had to step on it, and the numbers would inevitably depress me, not make me happy that the program was working.

I took it out to the trash can in the backyard, and I opened the lid and threw the scale away.

As soon as I closed the lid, I felt so relieved.

Fuck you, I said to the scale. *I have control of my life now.*

That was the biggest step to my recovery, but just like my addiction to drugs, my addiction to the scale is always there. I was able to complete that first hundred-miler, using the weight I gained before the race. But officials at hundred-milers make you weigh yourself before a race so they can monitor your body during the race. If you lose too much weight, they will put an IV in you or even pull you.

It was hard looking at those numbers on the scale before those races. It still felt weird. It still felt strange. But it felt right.

Now I just go by how I feel. Some days I eat more, and other days I eat less.

Chapter Eleven

Running the Race I Shared with My Father

In 2000, I got into Western States and immediately thought of my father. This was the race that my father pointed out to me when I was a bratty teenager. Now I would actually be running it. It was as if he led me to this moment and would be running it with me.

By that time, Western States would be my third hundred-miler. Despite all the pain it took to finish the Rocky Raccoon, I was enthralled with being an ultrarunner and the way it made me feel to finish a race. Sometimes you'll hear runners say achieving something like that is "better than drugs," but in my case, it was true. I no longer needed drugs to be happy or stable. My life was better than it had ever been.

I completed that twenty-four-hour run and began to look for my next hundred-miler. My thoughts turned to Western States both because of my father and because of the prestige of it. Western States is probably comparable to the Boston Marathon in terms of renown.

The Western States Endurance Run in Squaw Valley, California, is one of the four Grand Slam hundred-milers, meaning that it is one of the oldest and most prestigious ultra races in the US, one which all serious ultrarunners aspire to run. It was, by many accounts, the race that made people believe that humans could survive running a hundred miles in the first place.

Western States was a horse race first before it became a human racing event. It was the Western States Trail Ride, but in 1973, Gordy Ainsleigh's horse pulled up lame at the twenty-nine-mile checkpoint, and he was thus disqualified. A year later, he joined the horses on foot, to see if a person could complete the course. He completed it in twenty-three hours and forty-two minutes, just under the twenty-four-hour time limit allotted for the horses. In 1976, Ken Shirk become the second runner to complete the course. The first official Western States Endurance Run started in 1977 when sixteen runners signed up for it. Only three finished it, and only one finished in the twenty-four-hour time limit. They began to give runners thirty hours to finish. The next year, the run took place without the horses, as its own event.

So I was excited to run it not only because it was the race that inspired my dad, but because it was elite. It was, in many ways, *the* hundred-miler. It was the original, and it was still considered the most prestigious.

As a result, many ultrarunners wanted to run it, even back in 1999, and so the race held a lottery to determine who got to do it. Yes, people actually compete for a chance to run a hundred miles. I didn't want to enter another hundred until I found out in December whether or not I got in, nine months after finishing my first hundred. So during that time, I occupied myself by running all kinds of ultramarathons. I had a special ability to recover from the races even faster than many other ultramarathoners, and I couldn't get enough of them. They were not my drug, but they got me through the week. I was gone almost every weekend.

I was thrilled to get into Western States, and that's what led me to meet my first real training partner, Mike Palmer.

We were running the same pace at the American River 50 Endurance Run, and so we began talking. This is pretty common during ultras, as you're on your feet for hours and hours. You have to find some way to take your mind off the pain. Talking with someone is a great way to do this. I discovered that many runners were eager to help me through the tough moments because they were looking for someone to return the favor when they needed it. I made many friends this way.

I told Palmer that I'd gotten into Western States, and he replied he'd run it many times. He knew his shit: he'd run several hundred-milers.

"Where do you live?" Palmer asked.

I told him right away. This is not something I would share with any stranger, let alone some guy out on a trail, but I didn't think twice about giving my address to a runner. The running world is its own world full of its own codes and acceptable behaviors. Palmer was asking me my address because he wanted to meet up with me and help me train for Western States. He knew all the routes that would help me conquer Western States, and he would run them with me. Again, this guy knew his shit, and I was thrilled that someone was willing to teach me how to run the hardest hundreds in California.

Soon after, I'd meet up with him to train during the week, and on the weekends, we would travel to races together. This was a true running partnership, and it's an example of the bond you form with other people out there suffering with you. That unique suffering creates a bond that is hard to describe to people who don't run, or honestly, those who may run but chose not to run ultras. Many people can't relate to the kind of pain it takes to finish one of those races. The people were crazy but friendly and open and loving in a way I'd never experienced before from strangers.

But in Palmer, I found more than just a friend. I was thrilled to find a mentor.

Western States, despite its popularity, is not just a hundred miles. It's a tough hundred. I can hear the thoughts: Aren't all hundred-milers tough? Well, yeah, but this one was tough even by those tough standards. Western States winds through California's Sierra Nevada Mountains on the last weekend in June, starting at the base of the Squaw Valley ski resort (the start is up a ski hill) and finishing on the track of Auburn's Placer High School in Auburn. There's snow on the highest points at times, but the valley holds some of the hottest locales on Earth, with temperatures frequently reaching over 100 degrees. Over the course of the race, participants run up eighteen thousand feet and down twenty-three thousand.

But I didn't care that it was hard. I'd finished two hundred-milers already, one of them with my feet covered in blisters. I was starting to love not only ultrarunning itself, but also the history of the sport and the people such as Palmer who formed its small but intense community.

Western States also meant a chance to show my mom what I'd become, to show her a member of the community that I'd become. She hadn't yet seen me finish a hundred-miler. I wanted my mother to see me run around the track and have that moment, that proud instance that would come from finishing the most prestigious hundred-miler in the world. I wanted to hug my mother and show her how far I'd come. Western States was thus both the pinnacle of my racing career so far and another chance to make my mom proud.

At the race expo the night before, the general feeling was much different than any race expo I'd attended before. I felt like I was at the Super Bowl of hundred-milers. I looked around in awe as I spotted fellow vegan Scott Jurek and Ann Trason, a badass woman who beat almost all the guys and had won the women's race fourteen times before. But then I saw Gordy, the man who started it all by winning the first hundred-miler. It was amazing.

I checked in, got weighed, and felt a mixture of excitement, nervousness, and fear. But I had a big grin on my face the whole time.

Oh my God, I thought. *This is real. This really is going to happen. This was it.*

The next morning, I gathered around all my new friends, shivering in the chilly mountain air that we'd be begging for in a few hours, feeling nervous and emotional. I thought of my father, who would run the race with me in spirit, and my mother, who was waiting for me at the end, and this brand new community that was now a big part of my life. And then the gun went off, and I took off like a rocket.

I hiked to the top peak of Squaw Valley, since running up a ski hill is not a good way to start a hundred miles. Everyone was walking anyway, but I had a hard time trying to control the burning energy that was begging to be released. When I got to the top, I looked around, saw the downhill, and started hammering it.

I talked to another woman as I pounded the course. She'd already completed the race once before and warned me not to push too hard in the beginning. I'd heard that before, but I still had a hard time listening. I was too excited for the finish.

But the problem is, again, a hundred miles is a long way. Excitement can only carry you so far.

When I entered the canyons, the cool mountain air left in a hurry, chased away by the heat that rose from the cracks in the earth ready to seemingly bake my brain. The dust rose up from the ground and entered my nose and my eyes, caking over my sweaty body. In no time, I was the filthiest I'd ever been in my life. I blew snot rockets almost every minute in an attempt to get the dust out of my nose.

It was dry, hot, and brutal, and I tried to drink a lot of water so I didn't get dehydrated. But the water started sloshing around in my stomach.

This is part of the reason why it is nearly impossible to feel good all the time in an ultramarathon. If you don't drink anything, you won't finish for sure. But if you drink too much, or even just a little too much, your body can't absorb all of it because of the strain you're putting it through. That happened to me as my stomach turned into a tide pool and started rebelling in the dusty, hundred-degree heat.

I tried to find ways to battle the heat since I couldn't drink it away. I put ice cubes in my hat and bra and dunked a bandana whenever I found a creek and wrapped it around my neck. Other runners did the same. I came across one guy who was just lying in the water as if he were dead. The heat was a killer, and my stomach was taking the brunt of it.

As I climbed through the canyons, I quickly figured out that this was the hardest thing I'd ever had to do in my life.

But there were moments that made it fun. At the top of one section, a spectator was handing out popsicles. At another pass, one of the few times places where spectators were present on the course, there was a big, party-like atmosphere. And about halfway through the race, there was something I had to do.

About halfway through the race, I pulled an upside-down crucifix out of my shorts, a relic of my Goth days to prove to myself that I was a new person. I held it in my sweaty palm and looked out at the river as the bridge swayed. I honestly believed part of the reason I struggled was because of the crucifix. It symbolized such a negative time in my life.

I made a promise to myself that I would continue to strive towards being the best person I could. I didn't need symbols to continue to prove to myself that I was a new person. I knew I was. I tottered on my feet as I held it over my head and pitched it into the river. And then I took off. I felt better instantly.

At least, I felt better for a while. These introspective moments picked me up, but soon it faded into hours of solitude, with just myself and the dust and the heat. As night approached, I was in trouble. I was tired and hot and struggling to keep in fluids. I was also starting to feel sleepy. I would need someone to help me through it. Fortunately, I had a pacer.

Many hundred-mile races allow runners to have a pacer after, say, running fifty miles of the course. The best pacers are your saviors along for the ride.

Back then, there was no Facebook, so it was hard to find pacers who could get you to the finish line without being "in the know." This is why Mike Palmer was so valuable as a mentor: he seemed to know everyone who ran these races. And through Palmer, I met Ian. When I met him, Ian looked ancient to me. I wondered if he could keep up with me. But as I talked with him, I learned he'd finished the race ten times, all of them under twenty-four hours, an amazing achievement. He would be a valuable ally.

I was facing considerable obstacles to the end. My stomach was angry and expelling anything I put into it. I hadn't yet learned how to stay awake all night. I was also exhausted and would occasionally rest my heavy eyes, while Ian kept pushing me harder and harder to stay on my feet. I felt like a turtle, if turtles could run and get diarrhea.

All hundred-milers have cutoffs, generally at aid stations. A runner has to reach these points by a certain time or else be forced to stop.

You don't have to run fast to finish a hundred-miler, but you do have to be steady. You may only average four miles an hour, just a little faster than a quick hike, but you have to do that over mountains and all the rocky terrain that comes with them through the night and some of the worst heat you'll ever experience. It's not easy.

As Ian and I descended a steep section, I saw a group of runners just hanging out. *Why were they all just hanging out and laughing*, I thought, *and I'm over here suffering and dying.* I yelled at them to stop laughing, which made Ian look at me funny.

"Are you okay?" he asked in a tone that seemed to suggest that he was really concerned.

I looked at the group of runners again and saw that they weren't there. I was imagining them.

And then Ian grabbed me as I fell to the ground. I had fallen asleep on my feet. I began slapping myself in the face to stay awake, and Ian pulled out a NoDoz.

By this point in my running career, I had no qualms about using things like NoDoz pills to stay awake, but I regretted taking it almost right away. My stomach ached, feeling as if I had eaten rocks, and I had to go to the bathroom all the time now, not just sporadically. It woke me up, but my stomach, and my system, went from bad to completely trashed.

The cutoffs loomed as I went through one aid station after another, barely missing the horns sounding that meant your race was over.

The sun was starting to rise, but I had a hard time moving, and Ian didn't know what to do. I didn't either. I'd never had to worry about a cutoff before.

"Push as hard as you can," Ian yelled.

I began to run for my life.

I started crying because I was in so much pain, but I was running as hard as I could.

I gotta make it. I can't get cut now. I can't. I can't. My mother is waiting for me.

Ian and I got to the Highway 49 aid station as the horn sounded for the two-minute warning. I got on the scale, praying that I hadn't lost too much weight. I passed—barely—and the organizers began to push me out of the aid station. I had no time to comprehend what was happening. They shoved me away from the station and the horn sounded again.

Did I make it? It was hard to know.

While I still ran as hard as I could, at this point Ian knew I wasn't going to make it. But I thought I still had a shot. I tried to think about my father and how fascinated he would be with me running this race. But mostly I thought about my mother. I wanted so badly to show her that I was different. I had proved it to myself, but I needed to prove it to her.

But soon, it was over. The horn sounded, and I missed the cutoff to the next aid station.

Only it wasn't over for me. I ran through that aid station.

I wanted to run around that track at Placer High School in Auburn to finish. I wanted my friends to cheer for me. I wanted to be a part of the people who had finished. I wanted to be part of that family. I wanted it so badly.

I made it to the track, and it was empty, for the most part, except for a large group of friends waiting for me, who had heard someone radio that I had run through the aid station. I collapsed and started crying when I got there.

Organizers were starting to clean up, and almost everyone was gone from the stands as I ran in, but as I crossed the line, my mother came down from the stadium. She handed me flowers.

"You did it!" she said.

"I didn't make it," I said, and explained about cutoffs and the end of the race.

My mother hugged me, and as we started walked back to the car, her soft side made a rare appearance. She said the one thing that could make me feel a little better about my bitterly disappointing finish.

"No matter what," she said, "I'm proud of you."

Chapter Twelve

The Long Walk

Like any good Californian, especially one in touch with the mountains and beauty that surrounded her, I kept a photo of Half Dome on my wall.

Ansel Adams, the famous photographer, snapped a photo of the granite hunk of rock in 1960 that became one of America's most iconic images. You've probably seen the photo even if you have no idea what I'm talking about.

Half Dome is a part of Yosemite National Park, one of the world's most beautiful natural places and a paradise for rock climbers, mostly because of Half Dome and the park's other infamous granite slab, El Capitan.

I had a frame of the iconic black-and-white photo on my wall for years. I don't remember how I got it, but I hung it on my wall because it, unlike my life at the time, was classy and cool.

The thing was, I'd never seen it in person.

When I was on drugs, I lost track of the poster because I lost track of everything in my life during that time. But when I moved back in with my mom, one day after my workout at the gym I walked by a thrift store next door and there was the same poster in a glass frame. I was so excited. I grabbed it and put it on my wall at my mom's house.

One day not long after, Kevin, who was still just my workout buddy at the time, asked me to go to Yosemite.

This was in 1994, just two months after I was off drugs and recovering from a life of patrolling clubs and concrete in the city. I'd heard of Yosemite; it was, after all, an iconic national park. But I'd never been, even though it was only four hours away.

I'd never been camping or hiking or, at this point, even walked on a trail.

My first real exposure to the outdoors was on the Alameda Creek Trail. I did my long runs on the trail because it had mile markers, so I could keep track of how far I'd gone. When I ran on it, it felt like I was really in the wilderness.

And as I continued to wash the drugs out of my system, I began to notice nature even more. One day, driving to the bagel shop where I worked then, I noticed the mountains. I looked at Mission Peak, like really looked at it, without the gray sheen the drugs put over my eyes.

Wow, I thought. *That's amazing.*

The drugs sucked the beauty of life out of everything. I was in a constant haze. That haze felt good, but it was hard to see life beyond it. When I got off drugs, all of a sudden, that gray haze was gone. Everything was so colorful, as vivid as a movie. Hell, it was better than a movie. It was real life.

So when Kevin asked me if I wanted to go to Yosemite, I was excited about the trip. We hopped in the car, and I was ready to see this amazing place that everyone raved about.

But when we got there, our inexperience showed almost right away.

After a four-hour drive to the park, we wanted to camp for the night, but we didn't have a reservation, and it was crowded, so there were no slots available. But the guy who ran the campsite was really nice and let us camp in this little grassy area on the edge of the entrance.

I had worn cutoff overalls and was already shivering. I didn't even have a sleeping bag, a headlamp, or a flashlight, so we turned our headlights on. Kevin struggled through it, but he somehow did get the tent up; well, sort of.

The night sucked. We were uncomfortable, freezing, and unable to sleep much. But as we got out of the tent the next morning, the sun rose, everything smelled fresh and clean, and the light began to reveal the beauty of the park.

I felt this peacefulness come over me.

Despite his inability to set up camp, Kevin knew Yosemite well, having been there a lot. So he began pointing out sights to me, and I was in awe, *oooing* and *ahhhing* almost constantly.

Then he told me that we should stop at an overlook. Sure, I said, gazing at the sights around me.

We stopped, I got out, and saw El Capitan. El Cap, as rock climbers called it, is a majestic granite wall with routes that challenged some of the best in the world.

And then I saw Half Dome. My hand went to my mouth.

There it was, the formation on my wall. There it was! *Oh, wow*. That picture had been with me for years, and now I was seeing it for the first time.

I was so thrilled.

I was in love.

At that the time, I didn't know that Yosemite would spark a love for the outdoors that would lead me on some record-breaking adventures. And I especially didn't know how both Yosemite and the outdoors would help me through my mother's death because, of course, she was still alive then.

At the time, I only knew one thing.

I knew I'd be back.

Yosemite gave me my first introduction to the outdoors, but I relied on my new running community to get me hooked on them.

I thought that after the first hundred-miler, I would slow down a bit. I had nothing left to prove. I had made myself into an ultrarunner by that point and the training for the next race would help me stay off drugs and force me to eat more. I didn't need to run races all the time.

But I fell in love with everything about being an ultrarunner, not just the races themselves or the good feelings they provided. I loved the races, I loved the courses, and I loved the challenge. But most of all, I loved the people.

My new running friends were all types of people. Mike Palmer, for example, was an administrative assistant for UC Berkeley. Others were judges, attorneys, CEOs, doctors, and lawyers, as well as bank managers, singers, musicians, and actors. Some of them were very public about their ultrarunning life, displaying all their belt buckles they got for finishing in their office, or proudly wearing their hats and T-shirts they got at races. But others led a semi-private life and chose not to talk about it with others. Not many people outside of our community understood what running ultras meant anyway. They couldn't fathom running a hundred miles. You'd hear things like, "I won't even drive that far." But all of us runners used it as an escape. There were a lot of former addicts in our group, but there were others who had difficult jobs or were going through breakups or just needed to get away from the stress of their lives.

I left every race with at least one new friend because, since you're out there for hours, you've got nothing better to do than talk. I would find myself saying the most personal things to someone I had just met that day.

Just as what happens in Vegas stays in Vegas, what you hear on the trail, stays on the trail. You can talk about everything out there.

This openness is how I came to meet Linda, and that is how I would spend almost a week on remote trails trying to break a couple records.

Linda McFadden was an attorney who later became a judge. Many people called her Judge Linda, and so did I, but I had another name for her, too: Crazy Linda.

The first time I saw her was at the Morgan Hill Marathon. I was in the middle of doing a lot of marathons in California, and this one was on the list. It was my second year of running, in 1997. There was a woman ahead of me, and I ran behind her or close to her for the last seven miles of the race. She was talking to everyone who came close enough pass her on the shoulder.

I overheard her talking to someone that she had run a 50K the day before.

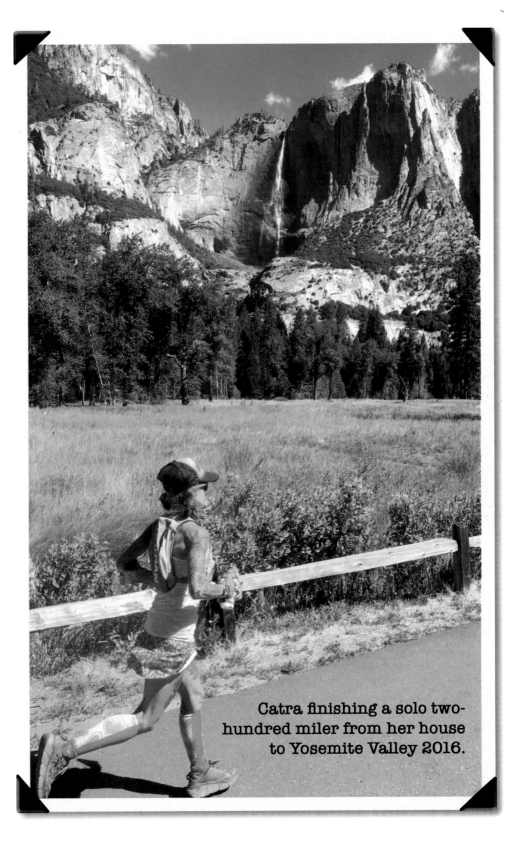

Catra finishing a solo two-hundred miler from her house to Yosemite Valley 2016.

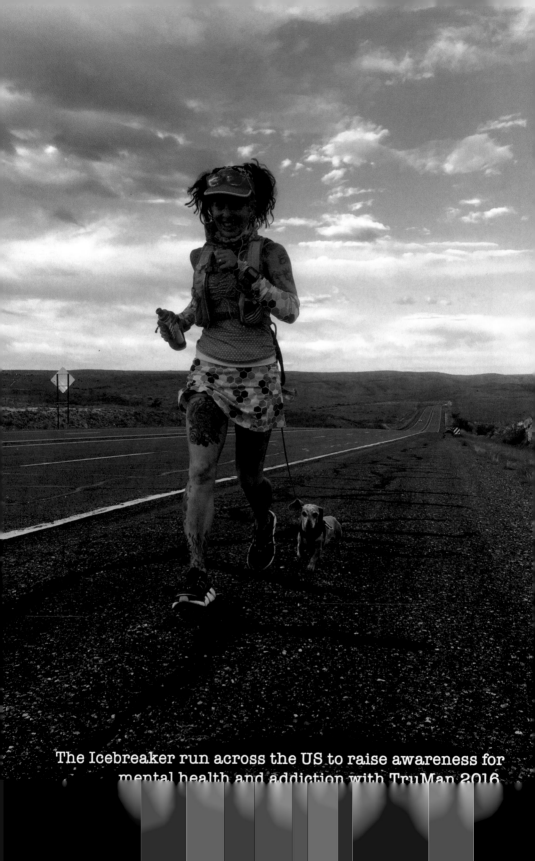

The Icebreaker run across the US to raise awareness for mental health and addiction with TruMan 2016

Catra and Charlie Engle running through New Mexico on the Icebreaker run in 2016.

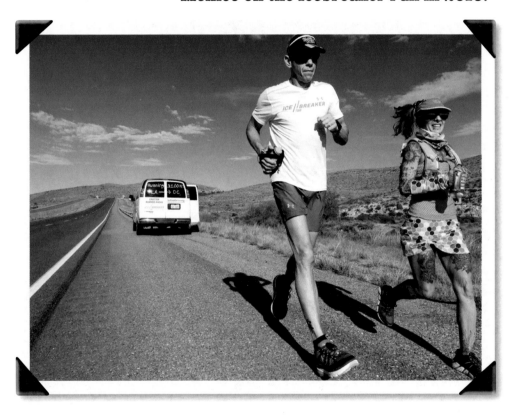

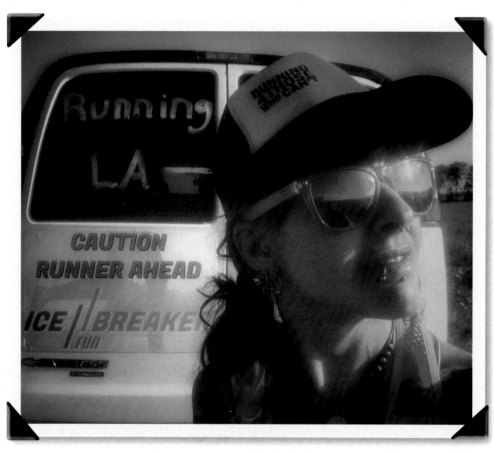

Catra on the Icebreaker run.

Team Icebreaker (l. to r.:) Catra, Truman, Sophie, Pam, David, Charlie, and Phil.

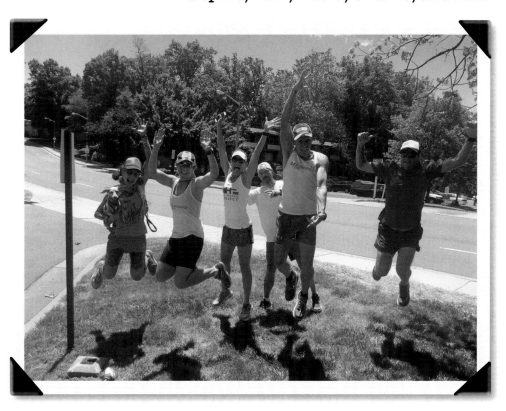

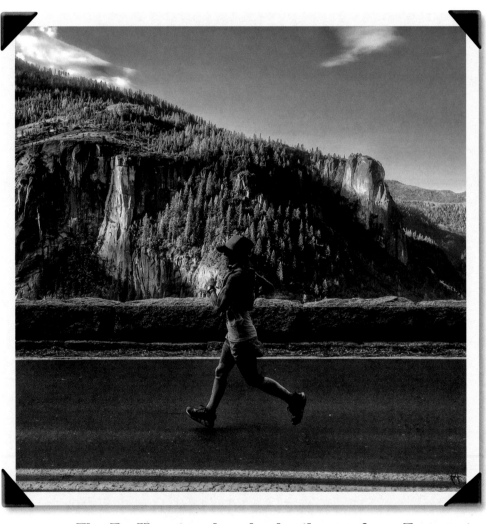

The FreYose two-hundred mile run from Fremont
to Yosemite 2016.

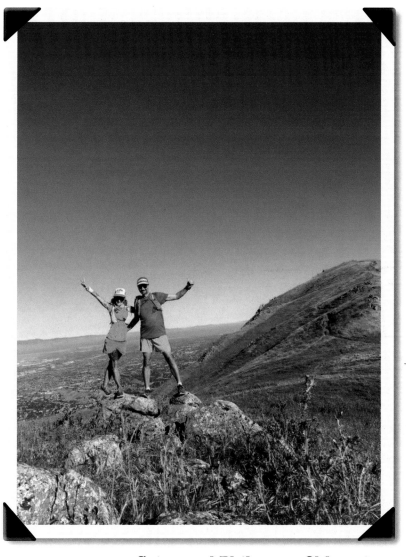

Catra and Phil on an Ohlone two-hundred mile run in 2017.

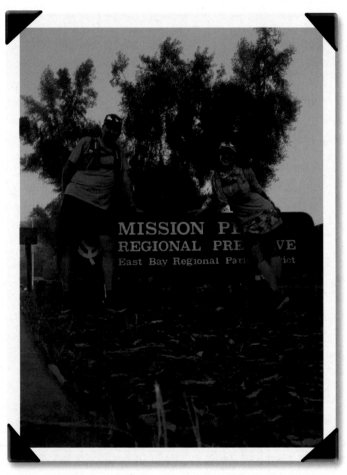

Catra and Phil on the way to the finish of
Ohlone wilderness two-hundred miler.

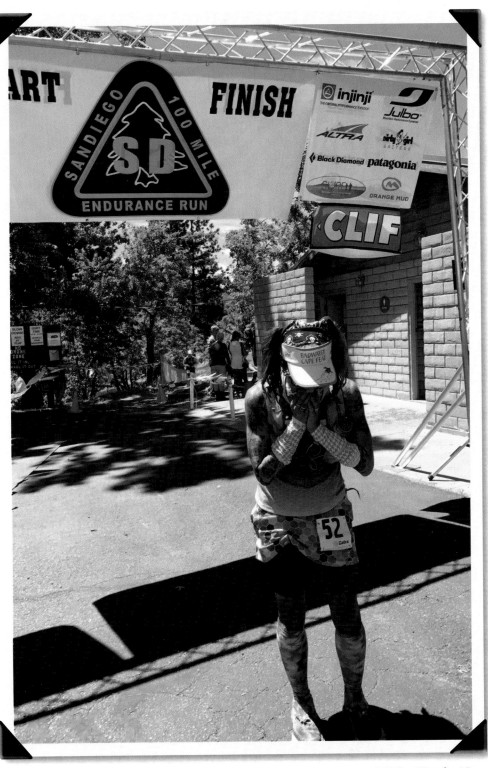

Catra at the finish of her tenth San Diego 100. She's the first female to finish ten times.

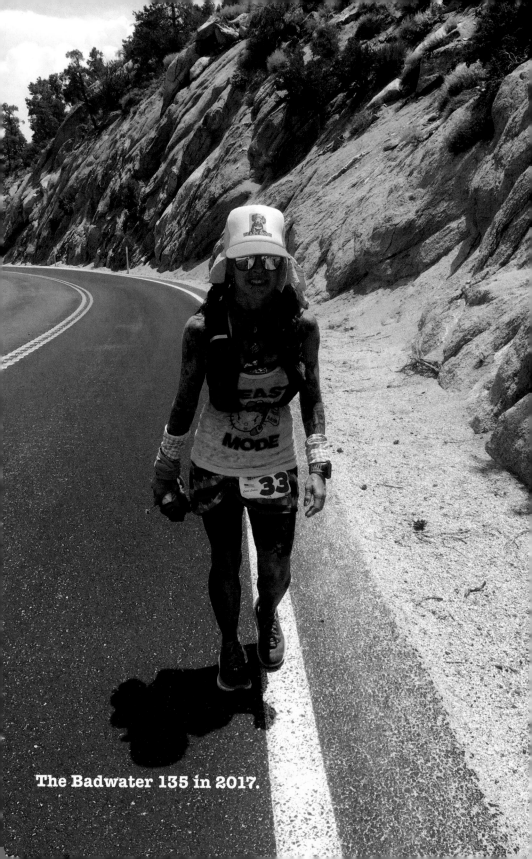

The Badwater 135 in 2017.

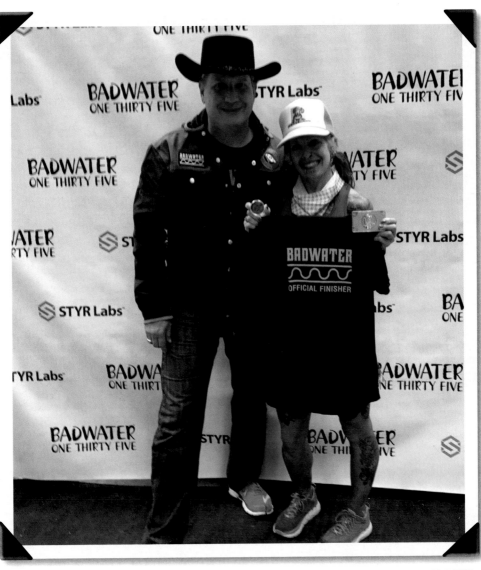

Catra at the finish of the Badwater 2017 with race director Chris Kostman.

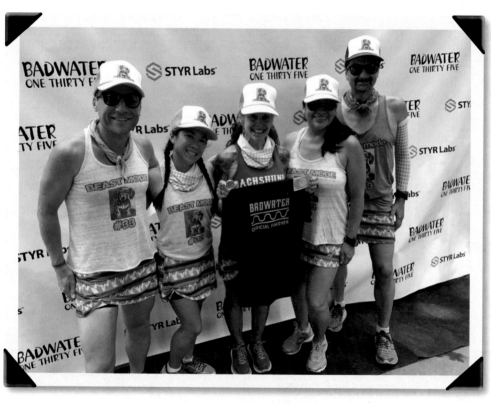

Catra Badwater crew: (l. to r.:)
Dave, Joyce, Catra, Gabriella, and Phil.

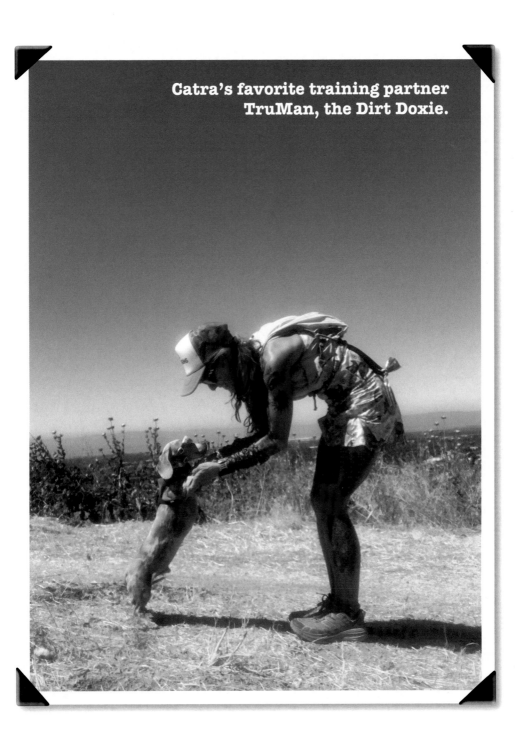

Catra's favorite training partner TruMan, the Dirt Doxie.

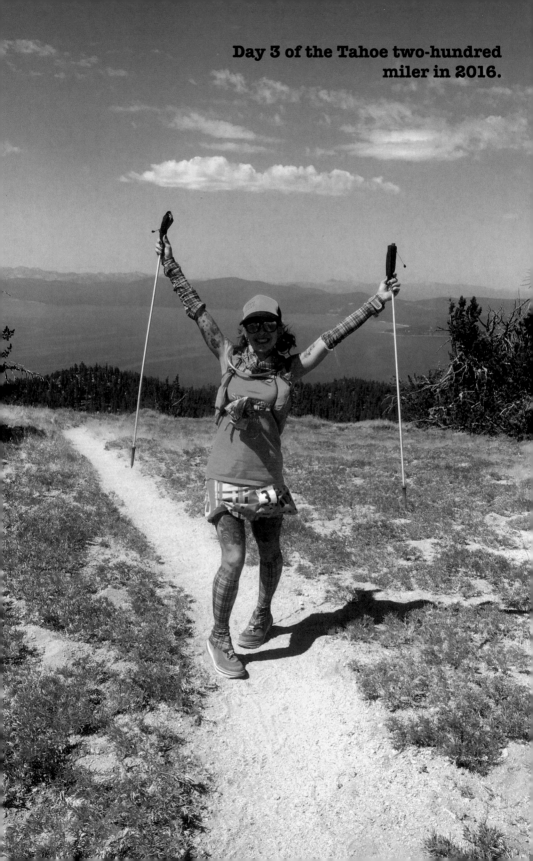

Day 3 of the Tahoe two-hundred miler in 2016.

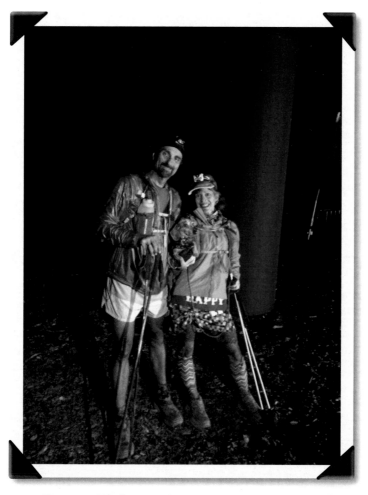

**Catra, Phil, and Truman at the finish
of the Tahoe two-hundred miler.**

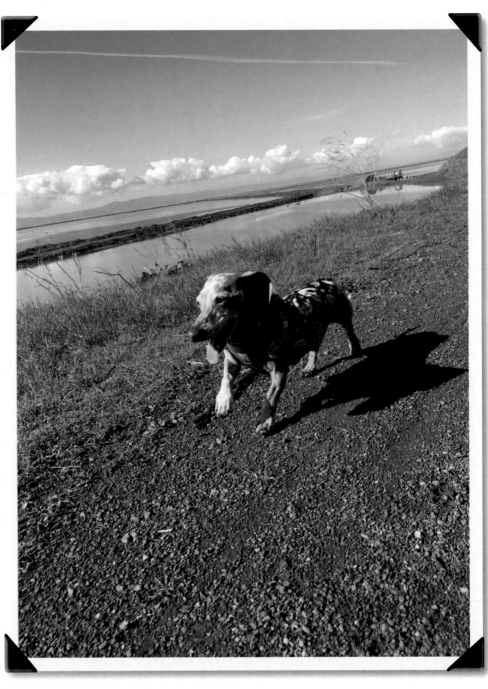

TruMan running Fremont 50k and getting a personal
record of six hours and forty-six minutes.

Oh my God. She ran a 50K the day before and now she's running this? Well, that was Crazy Linda.

At my first 50K, Linda pulled up beside me, and I told her I remembered her from Morgan Hill and expressed my amazement at her ability to run those long races back to back.

"It's no big deal," Linda told me. "You just train like that."

I saw her at another marathon a few weeks later, we exchanged numbers, and then started going to races together.

At the time, Linda was a prosecuting attorney, working on crimes against children. You can just imagine what she saw on a regular basis. She would talk about some of these gory details during races. Just horrifying stuff. I could see why she needed the release of ultrarunning.

Maybe because of the stress of her job, Linda was outgoing during the races. She was super friendly, warm, and talked a lot. Linda loved to talk. So it was no surprise that she booked a trip to run these amazing trails with Suzanne Krantz, another runner.

I met Suzanne through Linda briefly at the Way Too Cool 50K in Cool, California, in March 2001. I saw that she was limping a bit, and I asked her what was wrong. She showed me these massive, bleeding blisters, but she was smiling and spunky. I would learn that you never saw Suzanne any other way, even under the worst circumstances.

Linda brought up the idea of the three of us completing the Tahoe Rim Trail in record time. The trail was 165 miles long and looped around the Lake Tahoe Basin in the Sierra Nevada and Carson ranges in California and Nevada. The highest point was over ten thousand feet, and over the course of the loop, you gained and lost twenty-five thousand feet.

In order to get the female team record, what many runners call a Fastest Known Time, or FKT, we had around sixty hours to finish it. This was not an official race, but many ultrarunners would run famous trails, and a few of them tried to do it faster than anyone else out there. That was our goal. On paper, it sounded like we should be able to do it. We were able to run one hundred miles in a time in less than thirty hours, so surely we should be able to do 165 in sixty. It even sounded fun.

The trail forms a loop around the Lake Tahoe Basin in the Sierra Nevada and Carson Mountain ranges of California and Nevada. Today it is more like a superhighway of hikers, backpackers, and campers, but back then, it was poorly marked and barely finished in 2001 through volunteer efforts when we decided to try it.

Today, the Tahoe Rim Trail Association has a website that provides maps to download and gives descriptions of each area. It's almost impossible to get lost, even if you don't bring a map. But back then, it was hard to tell what the trail was and what it wasn't. Linda was good at navigating, and thank God, because it was a lot of route finding.

We hoped to go for the overall record of sixty hours. Linda, as always, had high hopes. I was just so excited to even be doing it. I'd never done anything like it before. It was not only a new challenge, which I loved, it was more like a new adventure.

We started out strong. The first day went well, and that night we were all fine, but Linda began complaining about her stomach. She always had stomach problems during races, and she started throwing up on the second day. As we approached sixty hours, it was obvious we weren't going to break the record, and I couldn't stay awake, so we all decided to sleep.

I'd never been awake that long before. Even during hundred-milers, I'd never been awake more than thirty-five hours. On this trip, I'd been up more than fifty hours straight and was hallucinating hard. I just didn't want to keep going. I decided I was going to quit.

After the nap, because that's really all it was, I told my teammates that I wasn't going on, and they told me that was fine, that I could stay with Linda's boyfriend, who was crewing us and bringing us supplies every twenty miles or so.

But that made me realize I was going to have to crew for them without finishing.

I had brought a T. S. Eliot quote with me: "Only those who will risk going too far can possibly find out how far one can go." I stared at the quote and folded it up and tucked it away and decided that there was no fucking way I was going to let them finish without me. I was making excuses, and the excuses were that I was sore and tired. There was no real reason I couldn't finish.

When the sun came back up, I started to feel good again, as I usually did when the sun greeted me during a run.

I got to the RV that signified the end of our run, I waited so all three of us could touch the side as per the record's rules. Suzanne walked with

Linda, who continued to struggle. We held hands, touched the RV, and then we scrambled inside and raced home.

We all had to go to work that day.

Suzanne had a painful and difficult personal life, but you wouldn't know that if you were around her. She was always smiling. She was a schoolteacher, a perfect fit for her.

I loved her energy. She was always so upbeat and positive.

She loved the outdoors. She loved the sky, the grass, and the lakes. She loved the mountains and wild creatures, both common and rare. One time, during a run with her and Linda, I was peeing and saw a rustling, brown bush about fifty feet away. When I stood up, I realized the bush was actually a bear. I screamed and dashed back to Linda and Suzanne.

"I JUST SAW A BEAR," I screamed, terrified. I would have peed my pants had I not just gone to the bathroom.

"Oh, you're so lucky," Suzanne said, smiling.

She loved every experience that nature could throw at someone because it was so different from her life at home.

She had gone through a horrendous divorce. She owned a children's clothing store as well, and her husband tried to pin a mental illness on her to make her lose the business. It seemed to work because she lost it and almost everything.

We talked about that during our miles on the trail, but then she would steer the conversation back to a bird or the clouds or the beautiful weather that day.

She was fearless too. She was this tiny woman, but she'd already been backpacking many times on her own. She didn't let the outdoors scare her. Instead, she allowed it to soothe her.

I was still the opposite. The outdoors still frightened me. I would need her courage desperately for our next adventure.

The John Muir Trail is more than 210 miles long, with an elevation gain of around forty-seven thousand feet. Linda, Suzanne, and I hoped to finish it in four days to beat the record of the fastest known time for a group, regardless of gender. But that was not the most daunting part about it for me.

The trail wound through the High Sierras, a remote backcountry and wilderness area known for its solitude. This made the Tahoe Rim Trail look like a suburban park. It was, in other words, the fucking wilderness.

I was still a city girl, and suddenly I would be in the fucking wilderness.

Linda planned our route, and once again, she had high hopes that were probably a little too high. Suzanne mapped out our supply drops. Linda's boyfriend, Jimmy, would once again help us out, but he wouldn't be able to help us every twenty miles like he had before. We were essentially on our own for much of the run.

We started the trip in Yosemite, and from there would travel to Reds Meadow, where Jimmy would meet us with supplies. This helped because we were able to carry run packs instead of the usual heavy packs you carry on a backpacking trip. That meant we could run at times.

When we started, it was 4 a.m. and already warm. Even with all of the trail above eight thousand feet, I knew it was going to be a hot day.

Everyone was feeling good, although the altitude was already starting to peck away at me. The only time I had run at altitude before was at Western States and the Tahoe Rim. I was huffing and puffing.

Ten miles into the trip, we had a big-ass climb into the High Sierra Campground, and those switchbacks went on forever. When we made it to the top, I was so relieved. We went into a store there for some snacks and supplies. We wouldn't get any more food until mile forty-eight, where Suzanne put some food for us into a bear box.

It got really hot after that. Linda thought we'd be able to make Reds Meadow in some ridiculously optimistic time, like sixteen hours. I guess that made sense at the time, given that we could run a hundred-mile race in thirty hours, but she hadn't counted on the altitude and the steep climb that was kicking our ass. As the day wore on, we realized that we had all our stuff at the post office at 6 p.m. We had to hurry or else we'd have to wait all night and into the next morning for it to open again. We would lose a lot of time.

It was also clear as we went on that Linda was having stomach issues again. I stayed with Linda once it got really bad, while Suzanne took off to try to make it to the post office.

It was getting later and later, and Linda was getting worse and worse. She began throwing up, and it seemed like she couldn't stop. At that point, it was late into the night.

At one point on the trail, we had to cross a log to get across a river. Linda's balance wasn't good at that point, and so she finally decided she could just cross the river on foot. I didn't think this was a good idea, but I let her do it because I was exhausted. She lost balance quickly and fell into the frigid water, at 2 a.m., screaming over and over because it was so cold. She got out and tried to get warm, and I just tried to stay positive for her, as we wandered around freezing, dusty roads, in the pitch black, trying to read signs that were unhelpful at best.

When we finally made it to Jimmy's RV, Linda was done. All I wanted to do was sleep. Suzanne didn't make it to the post office in time anyway.

We slept, and when we woke up, our plan had changed. We weren't going after any record. But we would go after the John Muir Trail. That was fine. We put on heavy packs and got going.

I was as ill-prepared as I'd been when I went with Kevin to Yosemite the first time. We had no tent, and I had a thin sleeping bag that you'd bring to a slumber party, not something to keep you warm at ten thousand feet in the Sierras.

I had packed for a running trip, not a backpacking trip.

The next morning, we got our gear together, got our food, and set out to make it to mile 105, where our next resupply was located. That was fifty miles away.

We made it thirteen miles.

I was exhausted at the end of the day, still feeling the effect of the night with Linda. We hiked up to a beautiful lake and hunkered down for the night.

Suzanne was enthralled with the lake and the air around her. I was terrified.

This was the first time I would sleep in the wilderness, other than a campground, in my life. The difference between a campground and the wilderness is the difference between a remote campground and your bed in your home. I jumped at every little noise that burst out of the woods. And because we were in the fucking wilderness, there were a lot of noises.

The night crawled along, and I tried to sleep but couldn't. I was too cold. It was freezing up there. Suzanne decided to let me use her bivy sack because she was prepared and had a down sleeping bag. I still tossed and turned all night. When the cold got to the point where I was shivering uncontrollably, I'd put my head inside the bivy sack and breathe heavily, over and over, letting the warm air wash over me. That would warm me for a bit, and then I'd roll up into a ball and twist and turn, but it was impossible to sleep in that position. When I got too cold and started shivering again, I had to do it all over. It was so uncomfortable. I didn't sleep much at all, and I desperately needed it.

We set out again the next morning, and I began to appreciate the area a bit. We climbed to Silver Pass camping at the lake there, and it was gorgeous. Suzanne was kicking ass. She trained at altitude, and was cheery and bright, as usual. She kept me going. It was the third night and we hoped to make it to Muir Trail Ranch, where our supplies were, the next day.

When we got there, it was great. I loved it. But when we opened our supply box, my heart dropped. There was candy and Skippy peanut butter. Two things that I still wouldn't touch. I had to dig through a leftover hiker box for something to eat, but I did find some things to munch on. Woods Creek crossing was our next supply drop, a long way away, and I needed to get something into my stomach.

As we made our way up Muir Pass, I was feeling good, and my pack wasn't as heavy as Suzanne's, who had the more typical frame backpack. So I began to run a bit. Whenever I did this, she was usually not far behind, but I kept going and going until I was up at the pass. I turned around, and then I didn't see her at all.

Where was she?

I took a look around and realized that I was alone, for the first time, without Suzanne's love and energy and support to help me forget how scared I was to be out there.

I started panicking, and then I started running.

What if something happened? I would be alone, by myself, in this vast area where every rustle seemed like it was a bear, ready to eat me. I had no experience and no clue how to survive out there by myself. I realized how much Suzanne had meant to me thus far during our time together. I realized how fortunate we were to have good weather because I didn't even have any kind of a rain coat or poncho. I mean, I barely had a sleeping bag.

I ran into a group of hikers as I headed back down the pass, and they asked me if I was Catra. I knew this was bad.

"Yes," I said.

"That woman you are with broke her arm," they said as I passed.

I picked up my pace. I was running as fast as I could go, even though I was already exhausted with my pack on. I finally made it back to the ranger's station.

"If you're looking for Suzanne," the ranger said to me, "she said to continue on without her. The ranger ahead was going to have food for you."

This was just like Suzanne, doing her very best not be a bother. She probably thought I'd want to continue our adventure in this beautiful place and not let something silly like a broken arm get in the way of it.

Ha. Yeah, right.

"I'm not going on without her," I told the ranger.

"Good for you," the ranger answered, sounding impressed. He probably thought that I was worried about my friend, but really, I was pretty fucking scared to be out in the wilderness, too.

Suzanne had started out hiking with an EMT, who was giving her Vicodin because she was in a lot of pain. It would take us a couple days to get out. Suzanne had her arm in a sling but would not let me carry her pack, even though she was in incredible pain. She was as tough as nails.

We slept that night with Suzanne sitting against a tree trunk and me stuffed inside the bivy sack. I didn't feel like complaining any longer.

When we finally got her to a hospital the next day, I met with Suzanne's friend and fellow ultrarunner, George Velasco. We found out that Suzanne didn't fall. Instead, she was just putting on her pack and her arm just broke. This was something more serious than a broken arm. Velasco walked out of the room after looking at Suzanne's X-rays, white and worried.

"She needs to get to her doctor now," he said.

Later, she would be diagnosed with malignant melanoma. The cancer had eaten through her bone and spread throughout her body, breaking her arm. The doctors gave her a couple months to live.

Sure enough, Suzanne defied the doctors and lived longer than she should have. She showed up to Rio Del Lago, a hundred-mile race she had won the year before, that November, several months after our botched trip. She was happy and positive, as usual. She was very sick at this point, but she showed up to cheer other runners on, even though she wanted to be out there herself.

A month later, she died.

For her memorial, some of her closer friends wanted me to speak about my experiences with Suzanne, so I talked about our trip on John Muir. I talked about how I was such a scared girl and how if this tiny woman had asked me to join her in the wilderness, I wouldn't have gone. But fate put us out there together, and Suzanne had this way of making me feel confident. By the end of the trip, even though we only spent a few days together, I learned a lot from her. She made me feel safe.

Suzanne was only with me for a short time, but she touched my life in a way that made me much stronger than before. I survived the trip. I would do many others in the future.

Suzanne passed away in 2001. In the years to come, I would go back to the John Muir and become a woman who needed the fucking wilderness because of the sadness I would continue to face in my life. Whenever I was there, I would think of her, since Suzanne is the one who gave me the confidence to go there in the first place.

I would always remember her in the wilderness. On our last day together, on the last thing she would get to do before cancer took over, while she was in horrible pain from the broken arm, she would look up at the sky and smile.

"Look at these clouds," she said. "Look at these amazing trees. We are lucky to be here."

Chapter Thirteen

On My Own

Here's the first thing you need to know about hundred-milers. They are not marathons. I finished most of the marathons that I ran in about four hours.

My mother had no problem going to marathons to watch my races. She knew what running meant to me, and further, it meant a lot to her, too, because she got her daughter back. So she loved to the races to support me. That is, until the races took longer than four hours.

Once I got into trail marathons, my mother would be there, waiting for me to run by, for most of the day. My first 50K took me almost seven hours to finish.

That was the limit: my mother decided she was done going to races. But even though she wouldn't be there physically, she'd still support me in spirit.

One morning, before my first fifty-miler, I found a little card from her, telling me how proud she was of me. So I left her a little card in return. This became a tradition between us.

By this point, I was running practically every weekend. I had completed many hundred-milers. My mother and I remained close. She was my rock. But I was always running one race or another.

Two years after the last race she attended with me, she needed some minor surgery for incontinence. She was getting older, but this was minor surgery, and her health was still generally good. There was no reason to worry about it.

So that weekend, I was running with a member of my new community, Wendell Doman, for his solo hundred-miler on Mount Diablo. He and his wife, Sarah, owned Pacific Coast Trail Runs, a company that put on trail races, and he wanted to scout the trail to see if it would be a good one for a new hundred-miler. I was going to pace him much of the way.

These were the kinds of things you did for each other. There were only a few people in the country, and really the world, who could run a good chunk of a hundred-miler with you. We all knew what it was like to do something like that. We knew the bad moments, and we wanted to help each other through them.

My mother, back from her surgery, had other plans for me.

"Can't you just be home this weekend?" she asked.

She was hurting and on pain medication. I saw my mother every single day, after work, and I honestly thought she was just tired and maybe a little loopy from the meds. It wasn't unusual for me to be out every weekend.

I thought my mother would be fine, and I also thought I owed the Domans since they always let me into their races for free and that they had reached out to me because they knew that I'd probably be one of few people capable of helping Wendell through this tough adventure.

But my mother's tiredness did worry me a little. I stayed the night at the Domans, and I called to check on her that night, and my uncle, who was staying with her while I was gone, told me she was sleeping. I told him not to bother her.

Wendell started his run on Friday. He was moving slower than normal and so even though I was supposed to come home Saturday, I didn't get home until 7 a.m. on Sunday morning.

I came through the front door, exhausted but eager to check on my mother.

I walked over to her room.

"Mom?"

There was no answer.

"Mom?" I said again, a little louder.

I noticed that her door was pushed halfway open.

"MOM?" I pushed open the door and looked over at the bed and noticed that she wasn't on it.

My eyes followed her off the bed to her body on the floor.

Her arms were extended, her eyes were wide open, and she was smiling.

She was obviously dead.

Seeing her was the most horrific thing that had happened to me at that point, even after a life with a drug addiction. This was far more paralyzing than my father's death.

I was so confused in that moment. Why did she have to die? She wasn't sick. Her health was still fine. I went numb and felt guilty.

I wondered if I had listened to my mother and stayed home that maybe I'd be able to get her to the hospital.

But as I screamed and cried, I looked at her again. She looked at peace. I interpreted that as she had seen my father just before she died. He was with her now.

My mother was very religious, so seeing her with the arms in the air, with that smile on her face, was a comfort. It would become a big comfort to me in the hard months that would follow. I liked to think that she was being lifted in the air by an angel. I like to think that angel was my father coming for her. It was an *I'm so happy* kind of smile. It made me realize that she was in a better place.

But still, it felt like she passed before her time, just like my father had. At least they would be together now.

I realized how well I had gotten to know my mother over the last few years as I planned her funeral basically on my own. I picked out her outfit because I knew what she would have wanted to wear. I picked out the color of her coffin because I knew what she would have liked.

While the funeral was nice (as far as funerals go), I decided that I would honor her memory the best way I knew how.

It was the same way I remembered my father.

I would run for her.

The Saturday after she passed, I would leave the run the American River 50 Mile Endurance Run. So that Friday afternoon, I left to go to the race.

Many people, including my brother and sisters, were flabbergasted I was going to run.

They called me selfish, which was probably true. But they didn't understand that this was exactly what I needed.

I needed to run, and think of her while I was on the trail. I also needed to be with my new running family. At that point I considered them as much my family as my actual family. Maybe more, if I was being honest with myself. There were a lot of ultrarunners at my mother's funeral service and the race director of the American River sent flowers.

Further, I didn't think that my mother would want me to not run a race because she had died. She was still a tough old lady.

I could hear her telling me to swallow the pain and suck it up. This wasn't just a scrape on my knee, but I know that she would be telling me I should treat it that way.

At the start of the race on Saturday morning, people were hugging me. They surrounded me with love and support. My running family was there for me. My community was there for me. I had found my place.

Once the race started, we spread out on the trail, running our own race, just as we should. I found myself alone, plodding along, after a couple miles. I felt lonely and sad. I began crying again.

"Show me a sign that you're okay," I said silently to my mother.

By the road, to my left, I saw a bunch of butterflies.

Huh.

Throughout the race, those butterflies seemed to follow me. Whenever I would get sad, I'd look back, and there would be a butterfly right behind me. I knew that that was my mother, telling me I was all right.

The next few months would be some of the roughest of my life. I felt numb, and I had to work through it. I couldn't just get over it. My eating disorder taught me that hard lesson. You have to work through the pain in order to recover from it.

The cause of my mother's deadly illness was an infection in her stomach. That's why she was in pain after the surgery. It was very sudden and was not something that anyone come have predicted, even her doctors. That unpredictability is one thing I leaned on as I worked through my guilt and sorrow over her death.

I expelled that sorrow on the trails. I was training harder than ever, and it seemed like every other day, I was crying out there, trying to work through my grief. Sometimes I would cry for hours.

What am I going to do, I would ask myself. *Why did this happen?*

When I wasn't running, I would hole up in my room. My sister, Patty, moved in the house and decided she was in charge of everything. That caused some tension in my family, but I didn't really care because I was in no mood to do anything. I didn't know where else to go or where else to live, and I had no motivation to try to find another place to live. Plus I just didn't want to find another place. As long as I was in the house, I was close to my mother. At times, I could still smell her.

I did have many people, most of them runners, tell me it wasn't my fault, and that always helped. Once I figured that out on my own, that really helped as well. But it took a while to accept that my best friend and cheerleader was now gone.

Probably the one thing that helped me more than anything else was I had a special event to train for. That same year, two years after my first try, I would run Western States again. I was glad I waited two years between attempts. This year would be the best to try it again. There were so many memories of my father associated with this race, and my mother was the only thing keeping me going when I was struggling so much on my first failed attempt. This time, I would think of them both throughout the race.

Weeks before she died, my mother looked at the date of the Western States race and noticed it was scheduled for her birthday. She was excited that I would be doing something that cool on her birthday. She knew that I learned about the race through my father, and she knew what the race meant to ultrarunners and how I ran it last time just so I could see her at the end. It was the first time she saw me finish a hundred-miler, even though I didn't officially finish it.

This time around, I would finish it, officially. I would kick its ass. And I would do it for my mother as a birthday present. It would be my way to make her proud.

I had trained extra hard for this race, I had great pacers and a good crew lined up from my running community that I now thought of as the only family I had left. I knew I was going to be strong because I was running it for her.

Just a few months after she died, I started the race with her picture pinned to my chest.

It was extremely hot once again. It felt sweltering out there. Around mile forty, I began to feel it. That was the first time I peed blood. I'd never done that before. It scared me.

As I struggled to run through the burn of what would be diagnosed as an angry bladder infection, I began to imagine in my head that my mother was alive and waiting for me at the finish. I had learned how to play tricks on myself in order to finish a hundred-miler.

The heat alone was enough to help me dream up an alternate reality where my mother was still alive, but the pain from the infection was there, too, all to ready to assist. I would deal with bladder infections throughout my running career after that point.

Every time I peed, it felt like someone had lit a fuse and stuffed it in my belly.

I ran into Gordy in the middle of the race, and by this time, he was a friend of mine, not just a hero. He could see that I was in pain, and he bent over me and performed some kind of magic on me. Gordy was kind of a weird dude, but you'd have to be to be essentially the first to try a hundred-mile race, right? He chanted over me a bit.

Surprisingly, against all expectations, whatever he did, it seemed to work for a while. The pain went away for a bit.

At mile sixty-two, I picked up my pacer, Jim, my older, retired training partner whom I had befriended during my marathons. He told me he would get me some cranberry juice to drink for the infection.

Aside from the pain of the infection, the 100-degree heat, and the weariness that comes when you've run close to seventy-five miles, I was feeling pretty good. That's how ultramarathons go. You don't finish them by feeling good. That's impossible. You finish them by limiting the negatives and keeping a good attitude about them when they inevitably happen.

At about mile eighty-five, we were in a good stretch of downhills and the pain was staggering. I was walking, and even though I had made good time throughout the race, I was beginning to wonder if I would make it to the finish again. At this point, the jarring of going downhill hurt so much that it felt like someone was stabbing me with a hot dagger just above my crotch. It was the most painful burning I'd ever felt. I couldn't stop crying. I was on a pace for twenty-seven hours, so I had a cushion, but even then, I really didn't know I could move another fifteen miles.

And then I thought of my mother.

I thought of my mother as the pain seared through my system. I kept thinking of how lucky I was to have her as a mother. I wished I could turn back time and show my appreciation for her taking back all those years that I was a brat and a drug addict.

But I knew she was waiting for me at the end. If I finished, she would come back to life.

I would have to be tough like her.

I thought that the infection burned whether I was walking or running. So why not fucking run?

I started running. I pushed the pain aside and wiped away the tears and started running hard at mile ninety-two.

"Whoa," the other runners said to Jim as he ran with me. "What did you give her?"

"I don't know," he mumbled as he tried to keep up.

At Highway 49, the chaotic rest stop that signaled to my last pacer that I probably wasn't going to make it last time, I started flying. Jim tripped on the trail and ripped a gash in his knee.

"Keep going!" he yelled. "Don't worry about me!"

My mother was going to be there at the end for me. My body was crying out with each step, and the hot dagger remained stuck in my bladder and I just kept passing people. I didn't see anyone around me. I didn't even know where I was. All I could see was the finish.

My life will now be different, I thought. *She will be alive, and you will have all this time with her.*

I saw the track and I charged around it in a dead sprint.

I finished, but where was my mother? I looked down at my chest, and I saw her photo.

And then it hit me. She wasn't there.

She wasn't ever going to be there again.

She wasn't coming back.

She was only there in my heart, but she wasn't there for me any longer.

I collapsed, sobbing. I sobbed for my father, for my mother, and for how lost I felt. I had no energy. I just felt empty.

I tried to drown the pain and the emptiness with race after race after race. I began to get a reputation. I was not only an ultrarunner now, but I was also getting a reputation as an ultrarunner known for doing epic shit. I began to think about doing things that not many people could do. And I did them because I felt lost.

Because I felt lost, I stopped eating again. My eating disorder, like my former drug addiction, was always there, ready to strike when I was weak.

I didn't want to be that person again either.

I didn't want to be anorexic.

I didn't want to be a drug addict.

I would need to find myself. I was in my thirties, lost, and again turning to laxatives to try to stop the gnawing at my soul.

I would need a place where I would find love. I would need a place where I discover how I could run not just for twenty-four hours, but for many days in a row, what the ultrarunning community calls fast packing. I would need a place that would give me an identity and a life for myself, one outside of my parents, and a place where I would rely on my ultrarunning family to show me how to do that.

I would head to Yosemite.

Chapter Fourteen

Yosemite: My Second Home and a Chance at a New Life

After my mother passed, I turned to Yosemite for solace. The wilderness and the peace it offered called to me. I still didn't feel completely comfortable in the wilderness yet, but using Suzanne's memory and inspiration, I knew it was the right place to help me get past the pain of my mother's death.

Yosemite calls to many others as well, and perhaps it is best known for being a Mecca to climbers for its big rock faces. Half Dome and El Capitan are not only beautiful formations, but they contain some of the best rock climbing routes in the world. I didn't really know this then. I was there to run. I just thought the rock climbing guys were kind of cute.

Most of the climbers stay in Camp 4, which is known as the unofficial climbing camp in Yosemite. I would usually stay in the nearby Camp 5 when I was doing my long training runs.

As a result, I would see the same group of guys in their rock-climbing gear. I would go on my long run and come back, and they would be taking their gear off for the night.

After a while, they began to ask me where I was all day, and I'd answer that I had run forty miles.

"Forty miles? Whoa. Dude." *Yep, I was legit.*

Once I earned their respect, they seemed to enjoy showing me all their gear. I would pick through their gear and ask what's this, and what's this, and what's that, and what are those ropes for, etc. It all began to pique my interest. Maybe, I thought, I could join these cute guys on those rock faces.

I would get the opportunity to do that thanks to Leo Lutz.

I met Leo at the Massanutten Mountain Trails 100 Mile Run in Virginia in 2002. We ran more than half the race together, mostly because I mentioned that I lived in California. Leo was obsessed with climbing, and so he not only knew about Yosemite, he was planning to come out and climb later that summer. We thought of a trip where I could go rock climbing with him and he could go running with me. Leo suggested that I climb Half Dome with him. He thought I could do a route called Snake Dike. We left the course as friends and exchanged phone numbers.

Leo gave me a list of what I would need and I went into Sunrise Mountain Sports in Livermore to buy the necessary equipment. It was the only place within driving distance where I could find a rock climbing shop. I gave a staff member my list. I needed a helmet, a belay device, a nut tool, and a harness. I told him I was going to climb Snake Dike.

"So you're getting all new equipment?" the guy asked me. Yes, I told him, I'd never been climbing before.

"You've never climbed before?" the guy asked. "And you're going to climb Snake Dike?"

The guys in the camp had said I could do it. The thing was, they seemed to base that on the fact that I could run a hundred miles. "You've run hundred miles," they said to me. "You're badass."

"I've run hundred miles," I told the guy. "I think I can do this."

"No way," the sales clerk replied.

Wait. Didn't he know I was badass?

He did sell me the equipment, and then he gave me, for free, some warning about the route. I took heed, picked up Leo, and headed out to Yosemite. We did a twenty-mile run, and then in the parking lot, Leo went through what we were going to do: how to belay, how to use the rope, etc. It was all new to me. The other climbers in camp were happy to show me their equipment, but that didn't mean I knew how to operate it. The next morning, we got up and began hiking up to the base of the climb.

We began going over cliffs and ledges, and I looked down.

It was a long, long way down.

Oops.

I quickly had a panic attack and started bawling. *This is what rock climbing is like?* The guy in the store was right. I was scared shitless.

We did make it to the base of the climb, and there was a group in front of us. The guy who seemed to be in charge turned to me and said that he recognized me from work. He said he didn't know I was a climber.

I told him I wasn't.

"Wait, you're climbing this route, and you've never rock climbed before?" he said.

"No," I said, "but I'm excited!"

Yep, I'm badass.

He shook his head and told me that he was an instructor, and that the people he was belaying had worked for a year to learn how to climb before attempting the route.

Oh.

That probably should have warned me to stop, but of course it didn't stop me from trying.

Leo told me then that the one thing I shouldn't do was drop the belay device, as it would help me arrest Leo in case he fell. It would make it much easier for me to stop him with the rope. It sounded pretty important to me.

I belayed Leo, who led the route until our rope was a straight line, and then it was my turn. I started climbing. I was scared as hell. But once I got on the stone, I just let my lungs go. The fear was real, but it added to the adrenaline I already had pumping through my body. I'd never done anything like that. It was amazing; it was fun; and, yes, it was badass.

I learned the lingo right away. "Climb on!" I said. "On belay!" I said. "Awesome!" I said. I got past my first pitch. I did it!

And then, as Leo was about halfway up the next pitch, I slipped a bit and let go of something.

Shit.

"Hey Leo?" I yelled up to him. "Remember that thing you told me not to drop? I dropped it."

Another climber called up that he had an extra one—climbers always seem to have a thousand pieces of gear—and he brought it up to me.

As we went on, I began to enjoy the fear that came over me as I was hanging from the side of a sheer rock wall. I trusted the rope and felt safe. I began to trust myself too. The pitches seemed to become easier as I crawled like a spider up the face. Climbers say this is when the route "opens up" for you. The puzzle becomes clear, and you can almost see where you're supposed to put your hands and feet, even twenty feet ahead of you.

Both Leo and I made it to the top of Half Dome, and it was an amazing feeling. I was in love with climbing.

It was what I needed to help me with the raw, lost feeling after my mother died. I had broken up with Kevin in 2000. He had become overwhelming, almost controlling, so I stopped talking to him. He didn't resurface again until my mom died. He came to the funeral, and then he started calling me again, but I still didn't want to get involved.

So I was alone and lonely, and after my mother died, those feelings intensified by a lot. The climbing, at least when I was on the rock, helped free me from all that sadness.

But now I had something else to focus on. I would continue to be a runner. Now I had climbing as well.

I bought a bunch of climbing magazines and began to read them, and I kept seeing pictures of this guy. He was one of the well-known Yosemite big-wall climbers. He seemed hardcore and badass, and there were a lot of routes that he was soloing on his own. I began asking people about him, and they would tell me that I was like a runner version of him.

He was also cute. His name was Ammon NcNeely.

In the spring of 2002, I was still looking to work out of the pain I was feeling from my mother's death, and I had been through the emotional

Western States race and was planning on running the Hardrock 100 in July. The course of the Hardrock winds through the beautiful San Juan Mountains in Colorado, which may be the hardest hundred-miler in the country. I was totally stoked about getting in, and I was training my ass off. In order to do that, I was running in Yosemite a lot.

Really, I was running off my grief, more than anything else, but I was also excited to run yet another amazing race.

I was crushed, then, when the Hardrock was canceled because of raging forest fires in southwestern Colorado. The year of 2002 had been a bone-dry one, and fires were catching all over the state. The governor made national headlines and earned the state's scorn when he said it seemed like "the whole state was on fire."

So since I was training so hard and spending so much time in Yosemite, I thought I would just run a hundred miles solo in Yosemite.

I invited some friends to join. My posse of course included Mike Palmer, my mentor, and a half-dozen others.

I started out solo at Yosemite Valley at 5 a.m. in July. I thought it was a going to be a hot day, but as we climbed higher, it stayed cool. I brought a light shell jacket because I thought it might rain. I met Mike near Tuolumne Meadows, an area with a campground one and a half hours by car away from Yosemite Valley. We had some massive climbs, but the group was strong. Everyone knew what it was like to suffer.

We could hear thunder off in the distance, and it got louder and louder, and then it started pouring on us and I started panicking. I had no clue what to do in a lightning storm.

"Mike, what are we supposed to do?" I screamed through the driving rain.

"I don't remember," Mike said.

The storm was suddenly right on top of us, which is sometimes what happens in the mountains. Storms aren't nearly as big of a deal in many areas of California where we ran, but in the mountains, they come fast, and they come hard; one bolt of lightning can kill you, especially above the tree line, when you're the tallest thing and almost asking for a quick strike.

Mike used to joke with me that he didn't want to be around me during a lightning storm because of all my piercings. He said that I would be a magnet for lightning bolts.

But with the bolts crashing all around us, I didn't know whether my piercings would attract lighting or not. Mike has a dry sense of humor, and he uses it frequently, but his jokes didn't seem funny any longer. Every flash of light from the sky made me scream.

We ducked into some trees, until we realized that those trees were the highest thing around, so we then headed back out in the pouring rain, with only our thin jackets to cover us and graupel started to pelt us. Graupel is essentially a light hail, which doesn't sound bad until you realize that there's more of it, and it falls faster than hail because it's tiny, meaning that sometimes it's more painful. We knew we would have to make it to the Sunrise Camp, the first step in a series of camps in the High Sierras.

So we ran our asses off, and we made it. The area is only open for backpackers, and it's super hard to get a spot. But the guy in charge that night was nice enough to let us hang out in the dining camp. Mike bought us rain ponchos because we were wet and cold.

Eventually the storm did pass and we were able to go outside. We started to run again, and I looked over to my left, and I saw a baby deer.

"Bambi," I said out loud.

I was close enough to touch it, but I didn't, of course. Instead I took a ton of photos.

While nature could be mean and vicious, it can also reward you with some special moments and beautiful scenery, all the time, as long as you respected it.

The rest of the trek was uneventful. I finished strong, and I was really happy that I accomplished something crazy like that and lived through it.

While I was not fast and I was not world famous, I was starting to be known for doing epic shit like running a hundred miles in Yosemite. There were maybe a handful of guys who were doing solo runs like that but hardly any women were at all. I was the first person who anyone knew who had run a hundred miles in Yosemite.

Doing stuff like that made me into who I am today. I didn't do these things because I wanted to be better than anyone. I just wanted to do them. I just wanted to run a hundred miles in Yosemite because I thought it would be cool.

I just wanted to do epic shit. And the next epic thing I would do was fall in love.

Because of my runs and the occasional rock climbing adventure, my name was starting to get traded around the camps.

I had been climbing for a couple months by then. I was known as the girl with the tattoos and pink hair who was running forty miles or more at a time. My name really spread after I ran a solo hundred miles in Yosemite. It really seemed to impress people.

Every time my name came up, people would mention Ammon as a comparison. At the time, he was doing tons of epic shit in Yosemite. He was known around the climbing world for first ascents, speed records, and solo ascents. Completing a solo ascent meant he was the first to climb a certain really tough route, a difficult accomplishment in the crowded world of climbing and it also meant he could climb difficult routes faster than just anyone. Solo ascents, however, were even tougher, as you generally had to climb the face at least twice, because you didn't have anyone to follow you and grab your gear once you were done. It was slow going. To put it simply, this meant Ammon could do things no one else could do. People thought that about me as well, and therefore, people mentioned us as a badass couple. But I had to meet him first.

I continued to spend a lot of time Yosemite, climbing and running, as much as I could in between work. I was there basically every weekend and it soon became like a second home. I believed it was for the best as I continued to grieve over my mother's death.

One day I was going to Yosemite to travel to the library to use the computers and I saw a guy on a bike outside the library. It was Ammon. I stopped the car and ran up to him, introducing myself.

"Oh, I know who you are," he replied to me. "People have been telling me I should meet you."

"People have been telling me I should meet you too," I said.

We exchanged phone numbers.

Later that day, Ammon came looking for me. He couldn't find me, but called me a couple weeks later. He invited me to his friend's house, and I invited him to my house. He was visiting a friend in Santa Cruz and I agreed to stop by. This was essentially our first date and we climbed together at the rock climbing gym.

He was a partier, which surprised me. He liked to drink and smoke pot. It made me a little nervous that I would try to join him and fall back, but I was still intrigued by him. He was happy and outgoing and full of life, much like some of the best trail runners I knew. He especially reminded me of Suzanne, who had died a couple years ago at this point.

I wanted to be like him. I wished I could be like that. I didn't want to be using drugs or alcohol, but I was so attracted to his energy and positive vibes. I loved it.

We started talking about my project. I wanted to run a hundred miles and then climb the Nutcracker, a classic, moderately difficult and popular route on the Manure Pile Buttress in Yosemite. Ammon told me he would climb it with me, even though it was far below his ability, and pace me twenty miles. We kissed over his promise to help me, and just a couple days after we met by the library, I instantly fell in love with him.

I was essentially this lost girl, sad, single, unhappy, and in mourning, and I didn't know where I was going with my life. He was waking me up out of my stupor. He made me feel alive again. He was the human spark I needed to really get back into my life.

A couple days later on the hundred-mile run, I got to mile sixty, and we were up around Glacier Point, after we had made it up and over Half Dome. We went into the bathroom to warm up a bit, and we were both there, shivering with each other. I had known him a week. He looked into my eyes.

"You're amazing," he said. "I love you."

"I love you too," I said.

At that moment, we became one entity, this amazing, well-known, badass couple that everyone seemed to envision. He was an incredible cheerleader and always had all our equipment perfectly set in order. He was perfect and caring and giving.

After that climb, we went through a brief but crazy courtship, and we were on Mission Peak together, two weeks after we had met, when he mentioned that we should get married. I agreed of course.

Yes, it was fast, but I was grieving, and I thought he was just what I needed. It felt so good to feel good instead of sad and lost. I was in love.

We thought about climbing El Capitan together and getting married at the top, but instead we headed to Vegas and didn't tell anyone. Less than a month after we met, I was sitting in a hotel room while he went to drink with his friends, waiting to get married.

It was a dream. It was amazing. And I was wondering what the hell I had gotten myself into.

It was too early to know that he was as fucked up as he was encouraging and wonderful. I couldn't have predicted the chaos that would follow. But I did know that, even then, sitting there with a cheap ring on my finger, that this was the wrong thing to do. It didn't feel right. But I didn't want to listen to myself.

I thought to myself, *Well, I want to get married, and I want to get married before I'm forty, and here I am, in my late thirties, in love. I might as well.*

I was in love. I was in love like I've never been in love before.

They say you will find this one person in your life where the fireworks explode in your head and you're just smitten. Every part of you just melts. Ammon was that way with me.

Well, at least in the beginning.

Chapter Fifteen

On the Road to Hell
with My Love

Every time I kissed Ammon, I felt butterflies.

That didn't change after the night we got married. He was the first person I'd been with who really made my heart flutter. I always thought that stuff was bullshit. I didn't think that actually happened to people. But with Ammon, it really did happen.

He sucked me right into his universe, and I let him.

And it really was a universe. When you were with Ammon, and he wasn't focused on climbing some super-hard route solo or something like that, you were in the center of it. He had a big laugh and a crazy heart, and he would make me crack up all the time. He would talk like a pirate, slipping into a character he referred to as the El Cap Pirate. He also could make me believe that I could do anything I wanted to. He was in awe over my running, and I was in awe over his climbing, and it showed. People often thought we were the perfect married couple. He was extreme, and I was extreme; he was crazy and I was crazy. We went together.

Wow, I'm amazing, I thought every time I was around him. He just made me feel that way.

It was also just fun to be with him. He was famous in our little circle, and I liked that. I hung around with other famous climbers—Dean Potter, Alexander and Thomas, who were known as the Huber brothers, Hans Florin—and when others would express their amazement that I knew these guys, well, I knew they were amazing climbers, but I knew them more as Ammon's friends.

I was still new to the wilderness and camping, but I was doing that with Ammon and the some of the most famous climbers in the world, so it was easy. He showed me all the cool spots in the valley where you could stay without being busted by the rangers. He called it "stealth mode" camping.

When I was with him, I could just roll through life. He taught me a lot of stuff like that. I had fun with those climbers. I had fun with him.

He was like a big kid.

I didn't even notice that others outside the world of Yosemite were shocked that I got married to this guy. What seems natural in the climber's camp in Yosemite may not seem that way to the rest of the world. The ultrarunning world was like that too. What seemed achievable, even normal, to us didn't seem that way to those outside our world. Sure, you could run a hundred miles. No big deal. Other people would look at you like you were crazy.

I guess it was probably strange to most people, including Patty, who shared our mother's house with me after Mom died, that we would get married after twenty-three days. It almost seems funny now that I wouldn't understand why she was so stunned when she had to meet this dirtbag climber after we were married and that he would be living with us. But I didn't think it was weird. The climbers in Yosemite's inner circle didn't think it was weird.

Instead, it was so fun.

I overlooked many of the warning signs, and I just didn't care because I was having too much fun in his universe.

But sometimes, that wild and crazy stuff can get to you.

Which is exactly what happened after he suggested I climb El Capitan for the first time.

Ammon turned to me in the climber's camp one day and said, "You need to climb a big wall. You need to climb El Cap."

El Capitan is the biggest wall of them all in California climbing. Even more, it is one of the most revered formations in the world amongst climbers. It was why Ammon and all his friends spent so much time in Yosemite. El Capitan made them famous because if you could conquer new routes that seemed impossible to other mortals, people noticed and word spread. Climbing magazines practically had stations camped out at the wall, ready to break the next big story.

Ammon was one of these renowned El Cap prodigies. He was just this kid out of Utah who showed up to Yosemite one day and shot through a solo route, easily completing the kind of feats that would eventually lead him to holding the most speed climbing world records on El Cap. (Soloing a route means essentially climbing it twice as there's no one to follow you to clean up your gear. You have to put in your gear as you climb that protects you from falls, and then when you're done scaling a pitch, you have to work all the way back down and remove the gear from the lower pitch, and then climb back up to the pitch you just climbed. It's truly badass.) And so, Ammon earned his reputation as one of the true badasses in the sport.

A year after we married, Ammon and a climbing partner, Ivo, were going to climb El Cap with his friend Bill and me. The route was really easy for Ammon. Ammon and Ivo planned to party their way up while we attempted to follow. But it was still El Cap. It would still be epic for me. And as game as I was for it, it would also be one of the toughest things I'd ever done.

The day started out fine, but the boys kept looking at the sky, and after a while, I figured out why. The forecast called for a big storm.

Again, Ammon and Ivo kept going because this route was no big deal for them, and I went along. But unfortunately, no matter how well meaning, Ammon's confidence was sometimes misplaced.

Bill and I were climbing below Ammon and Ivo. I was standing out on a belay, and there was a waterfall crashing over us. I was getting really cold, and I could smell and sense that the weather was getting bad.

At one point, Bill became freaked out with everything that was happening. The exposure was already an issue for him, and with the storm coming and the waterfall and the snow melt, it all became too much. He wanted to go back. The problem is, it's more dangerous to go down.

Ammon was trying to explain to me how to take myself on and off belay so Bill and I could both repel. We had to unclip and get to the other ropes to move down. While he explained it thoroughly, it was still over my head; it was a bit like someone explaining calculus to you when you've only just learned how to do algebra. I didn't understand it, and Ammon began to worry that something bad was going to happen if I tried to repel down the route myself.

So Ammon performed a fireman's belay: he tied me below him, and we were going to repel together, but as we were rappelling down, the rope kept skipping through the belay device. It was wet and chaotic and terrifying. At one point, Ammon pulled the rope and realized it wasn't tied with a knot at the end. Had we slipped at that point, we would have just slid off the end of the rope and fallen to our deaths.

When we transitioned to the next rope during our belay, the device wasn't locking, and we were sliding, and then abruptly, we were falling. The rope was attached to a belay station, but the role stretched into a J-shape, and all of Ammon's weight crashed against my body. The rope pulled on my arm and tangled it. All of a sudden I felt excruciating pain.

Ammon yelled at me to hand him my belay device, but I was hysterically crying in fear and pain. All I remembered was looking behind me as we were falling, and I thought my life was over. Here I was, against the rock, in intense pain, with the shock of a scare still streaming through my body. And I still wasn't on solid ground.

We had to finish two more rapels, and once we got down, we ran to a clinic in Yosemite.

The doctors there had seen the worst of what El Cap could offer. I was just another broken arm.

But that didn't mean I wasn't in for it. The doctor took a look at me, took an X-ray, and told me I need to have surgery and should get back to Fremont right away.

The doctor suggested some hardcore pain medications. I knew this doctor already because he was on the medical team at Western States, and I knew he was serious at the meds because he knew my past, but I still couldn't take his advice.

"I don't do drugs," I said.

The doctor looked at me.

"You're going to be in excruciating pain," the doctor answered.

He was right. Even after the surgery four days later, the pain was the most excruciating thing I've ever gone through.

That was just an accident. It happens. I had to sit out a bit for races, but I did manage to recover and start again. I was lucky to live through it and come away with just a broken arm.

But this would be the first sign that the fun with Ammon might end one day.

When I decided I wanted to tackle the John Muir Trail a second time, I hoped Ammon would come with me, but I didn't expect it. I knew that he was going for a speed record on El Cap, and he'd be there for a week or so. But when I told him after his climb, he decided that he would hike the trail with me. He was always excited about doing something new and fun.

We'd been married seven months by then, and this would be the epic couple's biggest adventure together.

I really wanted to finish the trail this time, since I'd never gotten to finish it after what happened to Suzanne's arm. I thought we could do it in seven days.

Despite all my experience up until this point, I was still naive about what it would take to finish the John Muir. I still didn't have good gear. I had a really thin sleeping bag that I gave to Ammon, and I bought a good lightweight one while we had two pieces of foam as our sleeping pads. We had no tent. And I packed a minimal amount of food. That was my biggest mistake.

We would start by climbing Mount Whitney, as the trail winds up and over the tallest mountain in the lower forty-eight states. Before we began, Ammon sat in the parking lot, getting high. That was his thing. As he was smoking, he dropped his pipe, and that set him off. But he luckily was also drinking an energy drink at the same time and was able to make that long can into a pipe. He was happy about that and, once he finished, off we went.

Minutes after starting, Ammon just went flying up the first hill. I was struggling a bit, as Whitney is more than fourteen thousand feet tall, which was high for me. Ammon was more used to the altitude than I was at that point. Hell, he was even smoking pot as he sped up the hill.

He was loving it, and it made me happy to see him happy, even as I was struggling. When we got near the top, we found a hut, and I went inside to lay down. I wanted to stay there, but we were on a mission to get some miles in—yet another mistake. We headed down in the dark and pushed pretty hard. By 1 a.m., I was so exhausted, I started hallucinating. By now I was used to seeing things in the dark: hallucinations are just a part of ultrarunning. But the altitude made them a lot stronger than normal. I kept seeing wiener dogs. Oskar had died by then, and I hadn't yet gotten another dog.

That was our first night. Pot, phantom wiener dogs, and huffing and puffing.

On the second day, after crossing over Forrester Pass and running into some snow, we hiked our way into the night, again, to get to the next pass to avoid camping lower in the meadows. I knew enough to know that I didn't want to sleep in the meadow because that's where most of the mosquitoes were located. We were climbing up into the next pass and were both so tired that we stopped for a rest and to eat.

I soon realized that Ammon was eating a lot. Like a lot. And I also realized that I didn't pack that much food.

That wasn't his fault. Ammon had just come off the wall after a big climbing trip, and he probably lost at least ten pounds up there in the week. I was well past my eating disorder by this time, but I still wasn't a big eater, but I just didn't expect Ammon to eat a ton more than I did.

He was hungry. I didn't know how to tell him to slow down on the food, so I just didn't eat much. He needed the food more than me. His energy reserves were low.

The problem, of course, is that meant both of us would be tested by lack of resources; Ammon as his supply of weed ran low, and me as I got more hungry. That's not a good mix as you walk and walk and walk your way into exhaustion many miles down a trail with mosquitoes buzzing all around you. Plus we were tired, and cold, and having trouble sleeping.

But somehow we did make it over Muir Pass, one of the checkpoints on the trail that offered a place to rest. We were just absolutely exhausted.

But we but we still didn't stop. Looking back, we should have stayed in a hut there. There we would have been protected from mosquitoes and cold. We needed the rest. We were going at least twenty miles a day, and even for us, that was a lot. We really should have stayed in the hut. But we were running really low on food, and so I thought we had to go on.

Ammon insisted we stop, but I told him then that we were almost out of food, and he freaked out. I calmed him down by telling him that we could make it to the next checkpoint, the Muir Trail Ranch, a wilderness ranch and a famous landmark on the trail. It was also a place that offered a community box full of food left behind by other backpackers. Backpackers had food shipped to the ranch and used it as a drop because they can't carry all the food they need, especially if they planned to hike the whole trail. The hiker box was full of food left behind by backpackers or by those who didn't collect their drops for one reason or another. It would be a huge help to us. We get more food that way. But that meant we had to leave the hut.

We were trudging along the trail again, with mosquitoes buzzing into small, thick clouds around our faces. I went to spray bug repellent on Ammon, but the top of the canister flew off and the DEET squirted him in the eye. I felt bad, because his eye felt like it was on fire. I've heard that stuff can blind you. That set him off since, at this point, we were hungry, tired, and irritable. And so we just started fighting about everything.

He kept snapping at me, and I didn't really want to fight back because I understood why he was grumpy. He was hungry. But he hadn't helped me prepare for the trip at all; he could have packed more food, and I was hungry too. So I started yelling at him. He called me a bitch, and I called him a fucking asshole, and he just took off and started running down the trail.

Now I was alone, and I hadn't been alone in the wilderness since my trip with Suzanne. As much progress as I made after my trip with Suzanne, the wilderness still scared me.

I began crying and screaming for him. I started running down the trail and screaming his name.

For fifteen minutes, I was crying his name when I saw a couple coming toward me.

When I asked them if they had seen someone, they told me there was a guy in the trees close by.

Ammon had hidden along the trail and was following me as I cried his name. That shook me up. It was fucked up and creepy.

But he emerged after a bit and apologized, so I apologized too, and we were able to walk again. But by this time, we realized how wrung out we were, and we had to stop again. We brought out our thin pads and tried to sleep in the cold amongst the swamp of mosquitoes. It didn't work. The bugs bit all night in search of our blood, and by this time, we were out of bug repellant. We shivered and yelped, tossed and turned. The first light of the morning sprayed over the meadow, and getting to the Ranch was more important than ever. We had to get food and more bug spray, pronto.

We eventually made it to the Ranch, where we found the scraps of food left behind by other backpackers. Ammon made quick work of the food, but he wanted more, real food. I told him that if we made it to Reds Meadow, a resort and packing station on the trail that sold the real food he craved, he could get a burger and a beer. So the next day, he had one goal: food and alcohol.

It was hard going getting there. I was exhausted and emotional, thinking about my mom and Suzanne. He kept having to wait for me to catch up.

But we made it to Reds Meadow. Ammon was so happy. He got a cheeseburger, fries, and a couple of beers. I had a salad.

So now we were both satiated and content, especially Ammon, even though I had no more money left. But that didn't matter right away because we were getting along; we even had sex on the trail.

The climbs, however, continued to be brutal and hot, and we were tired. We pushed pretty hard to get to Yosemite, and once we were able to see Half Dome, we pushed even harder.

We were dusty and dirty and hot, and we hadn't showered for a week. At this point, Ammon looked like the one with the eating disorder. He was as thin as a skeleton. We made it to the next stop, Tuolumne, and Ammon saw a bunch of his climbing buddies. He saw this as a temporary opportunity to return to his life of hanging out with his friends and climb. He wanted to hang out and drink beer and eat with twenty-five miles to go.

I wanted to leave. We stunk and I was exhausted, but Ammon insisted on partying for a bit.

We ended up leaving in the dark and had to sleep in the meadow again.

When we made it down to the valley the next afternoon, we'd finished the hike. We were happy but not elated as we should have been. He was starving, and so was I.

Ammon's brother, who was supposed to pick us up, wasn't going to be there for another day and my wallet was in his vehicle. Ammon wanted a sandwich. I told him we needed to borrow money from someone.

We got to the store, and I looked over just in time to see him stealing a sandwich.

"What the fuck!" I yelled at him. "No way. You're not stealing around me."

"Shut the fuck up," he whispered hard through his teeth.

It went on from there. We got into a really heated argument. He was pissed off that I said anything and I really pissed off that he would try something like that. That wasn't the kind of person I wanted to be.

We had just completed the John Muir Trail together, in a week, and it was pretty amazing to accomplish. It was something I'd always wanted to do, and after two tries, I'd made it, and I'd made it with my husband, the man I loved, the guy who gave me butterflies whenever I kissed him.

But that trip was the first time I truly realized that we really weren't the best team. But I was married to him. For better or worse, I was here for the long haul.

My suspicions that I felt that night in Vegas were true.

He was just a big kid—not an adult. And I loved him.

I was fucked.

My brain gave me the warning signs, but my heart ignored them. Ammon made that easy.

When we finished the trail, he told me he wasn't going to smoke pot as much, or drink as much, and that he would be around more and support me. I had a bunch of hundred-milers coming up that fall, and he wanted me to do well.

It was probably not a coincidence that he said these things in the fall, when the air started getting cooler, signaling winter's approach, and Ammon recognized that he wouldn't be climbing as much. We were married, so we lived together. He wasn't being devious. But I would learn later that he was following a pattern. He made all these promises, to make people happy for the moment and give him a place to hole up for the winter. I wasn't the first girl to hear these false promises or to fall for them.

Our relationship was still good at that point, however, and as the summer wound down and Yosemite began to lose its appeal once it got colder, I refused to back off, let alone let him go. He was too fun and spontaneous and thoughtful. I ran the Wasatch Front 100 Endurance Run in September, and he acted as both a pacer and my crew, and he did a fantastic job. He was really organized. When I got to the aid station, Ammon had everything all lined up so I quickly could figure out what I wanted.

I spent the fall running my hundred-milers, and he spent the fall climbing back in Yosemite.

We were still that extreme couple, the one I loved us being. While what happened on the John Muir had been a warning sign, my heart was full. I didn't want to listen to it. Ammon made that easy.

Come winter, when ice covered the climbing routes, Ammon stayed at home a lot more. I worked during the day at Whole Foods. I loved running, but running was not the only thing I had to do in my life. I needed be an adult and make money. But Ammon, because he was still a big kid, did not want to adult.

Money was tight, and I began to hound him to find a job. Ammon didn't want to work, and he had nowhere to go. He spent many days drinking and on the computer. In fairness, for some of those days, he was writing about his climbing for magazines, and he would get paid for those articles. But on most days, he would do nothing.

It felt like I was paying for everything and like he had no responsibilities. It still felt like he had no life beyond climbing. Ammon didn't even have a driver's license.

I get his desire to live off the grid. That appeals to the ultrarunner in me. But the adult in me knew that I couldn't do that. I once lived a partier's lifestyle and was, for many years, a big kid like Ammon. I was high most days, and I had the energy of a teenager when I was on a good high. I danced many nights. I hung out until daylight.

But I always worked, even then, and as much fun as it could be to be a kid, I always realized that you can't be a kid forever. Ammon didn't realize that, and it felt like I was taking care of a kid. It got old after a while.

I had bills I had to pay, and I couldn't just be in stealth mode, stealing sandwiches and camping spots in Yosemite. I couldn't just freeload the rest of my life. I'd never had more fun in a relationship, but the fun was fading fast.

Ammon could sense it too.

The thing was, the spontaneous side made him great and was what kept me coming back. He could go with anything. He could be creative and solve routes in rock that few climbers in the world could. He could show up in Yosemite and spend a month soloing a big wall on a super hard route. But spontaneity comes with a few side effects. Spontaneity meant you would have a beer at 11 a.m., or you would spend a week on a route, or you would hook up with a girl because it felt right. Ammon was married at nineteen, and he had kids. When I met him, he had a kid from one girl and he had gotten another pregnant. But I didn't know that at the time.

I thought I was different from all the other girls. I was married to him after all. I should have seen that he bounced around from girlfriend to girlfriend, and that's how he lived, like a kind, loving, and supportive parasite.

Then again, how the hell well can you know someone in twenty-four days? It took him longer to solo the route that brought him fame and fortune.

That's why it didn't feel right in that Vegas hotel room, and that's why my brain tried to overrule my heart.

It didn't work.

At least he kept one promise.

He did quit smoking.

Chapter Sixteen

The John Muir Speed Record

When I fastpacked the John Muir with Ammon, we ran into a couple hikers who mentioned that they knew someone who completed the yo-yo, or out and back of the entire trail, in sixteen days. I replied that I thought I could do it in twelve. Ammon, who was already exhausted during our seven days on the trail, shot me a look.

"I'm not doing it with you," he said definitively.

That stayed with me.

I wanted to try it and he just shut me down, without a second thought.

I was an ultrarunner, but I was also entrenched in the climbers' camp and knew that one of the accomplishments they treasured were speed records. El Capitan had basically been climbed by everyone who mattered, so the best way to separate yourself from the other top climbers was to do those routes fast. Ammon had a few of those records, and that's what made his reputation.

I decided I wanted my own speed record. I couldn't fly up El Cap, but I could push on the trail. I believed that I could push longer and harder than just about anyone in the country. It was time to put that to a true test.

Ammon and I made it through the winter, with him doing the occasional odd job and mostly me supporting us. As the summer approached, with Ammon back on the rock, I didn't feel guilty about taking a break to try to accomplish what I thought would be an amazing record.

I had a friend, an ultrarunner named Jeff Heasley, who wanted to finish the first half with me. I met Heasley earlier that year at the HURT Trail 100-Mile Endurance Run in Honolulu. I talked with him about the John Muir Trail and my desire to go for the speed record. Heasley wanted to fastpack it and agreed to go one way with me. I really wanted Ammon with me, but I figured Jeff would be a good consolation partner. I also figured that because he lived in Colorado, the altitude would not be a problem for him.

I didn't have a GPS back then—no one really did—and so I just went by maps. I calculated the amount of mileage I'd need to accomplish each day for twelve days—about thirty-five miles a day—and where I'd need to sleep, and I would push to these sleep spots. I had it all planned.

Of course, what you can do on paper isn't what you're doing on the trail. I would find that out quickly. It would, in many respects, be the hardest thing I'd ever done.

Jeff and I started and went at a fast clip to get the first twenty-five miles in. After just a few hours, Jeff was throwing up. He couldn't drink water. He may have been okay in the altitude, but I forgot about the heat.

It is so, so, so hot in the summer. It's basically a desert, even in the higher country. There is a store nearby, one of the few to serve hikers along the trail, and he continued puking. He couldn't keep anything down. We were not off to a good start.

Ammon met us at the store, and he told Jeff to take a couple hits off his weed. That would make him better.

Great, I thought, already tired of Ammon's constant smoking and drinking and how it was affecting our relationship.

In fairness, though, weed is known to curb nausea. Jeff took a few hits, and it did actually settle his stomach. Score one for Ammon.

On that first day, we were climbing up Donahue Pass, Jeff was feeling better, and I was getting more excited about this whole journey. I was attempting my own thing for the first time. I had completed many organized hundred-milers by this time, and I had done some fastpacking too, but this was my own trip, my own journey, and my own speed record. We did a major push of sixty miles in twenty hours. We were flying.

The second day we did a bit under thirty, and on day three, we did a hard push to make up some of the mileage we lost from our casual day of resting by only going thirty. We did three really hard passes in a row, and I was struggling up the mountains.

This trail wasn't just about mileage. I, like many of my ultrarunning friends, honestly could do thirty-five miles a day for twelve days straight without much of a problem. But this obviously wasn't just going for thirty-five miles and then going home to shower and rest. This was thirty-five miles with a pack on, up and up and up some steep mountain passes, hiking and running for hours a day, and then camping out, waking up, and doing it again.

When I struggled, I tried to think about my mother. I would pray to her to give me her strength, determination, and most of all, her stubbornness.

We kept pushing, and I used all of the strength my mother had given me that day. We went far into the night and I was just wrecked. Jeff and I collapsed into our tents, and I noticed my feet were hurting. I thought I was getting some blisters, but I decided not to worry about them.

That would be a big mistake.

A couple days later, we reached the top of Mount Whitney in five days, fifteen hours, and fifty-five minutes. Jeff and I said our good-byes, and I stumbled down the mountain, in the wilderness.

It hit me that I would be going out on my own, into the wilderness, from here on out. The previous year, when Ammon ditched me for a bit, I was so scared I was in tears. I really hoped not to repeat that terror.

The first few hours didn't go well. I took some wrong turns, and I started crying because of the time I was losing, plus my feet were really hurting. At midnight, when I finally hunkered down in my little tent, my feet were killing me. I took off my socks for a look.

They were blistered up really bad. There were half dollars on my heels, blisters coating my toes, and puffy patches on the surface of my feet.

My feet were worse than they were during my first, painful hundred-miler when I had to battle blisters for forty miles to finish.

I would have to do forty miles a day now, for a week, with these same blisters.

Mom, I thought. *I'm going to need your stubbornness more than ever.*

Every morning after that, I had a routine. I'd sterilize a safety pin, pop my blisters, and take two Advil. I covered them with blister tape. I would put on my shoes and stand up. And then I would cry.

By the second day on my return trip, as I was battling my own clock for a personal speed record, the pain was horrible. All I could do was hobble. Every step brought more tears. I needed a boost. Luckily, I got one.

A couple days prior, I'd ran into a hiker on a divergent path. He was doing the Pacific Coast Trail (PCT). But we chatted for a bit and during our good-byes, he gave me a name that stuck. He said I looked like a diva coming up on the trail and looking all colorful and cute.

Then he looked me over.

"You're a dirty diva though," he said.

It became my trail name. Dirt Diva it was. (Dirty Diva sounded like a porn name.) He said he would spread the word about me.

He kept his word. I started out on the trail that morning, in tears, and people began to cheer for me as I went by. I was easy to spot. I was the only filthy colorful girl who was hiking both ways.

"Dirt Diva!" they would yell. "You can do this. You're doing great!"

I had no idea what was going on, until I heard that the word was spreading about me on the trail. Some of my ultrarunning friends were talking about me, and that was enough to send the news down the path. When they saw a grungy, dirty girl running by herself who looked as if she was running on hot coals, with pink hair and a few tattoos and some piercings, they figured I must be the Dirt Diva going for a speed record. People wanted photos with me, despite my stench, and they were all in awe of me, which made me feel great.

I had to do this alone. The only people who could honestly hang with me during this push were my father and mother. I suppose Suzanne could too, of course, but my parents were on my mind for this trip.

Please keep me safe, I said to them. *Give me strength.*

I would draw on their strength and the strength of others.

I wanted to make my parents proud, but I wanted to make Ammon proud too. I thought that was sort of sick of me. Things weren't going well between us. I wasn't happy, and I sort of sensed that he wasn't either. But I still loved him, and I loved what he could do. I wanted to be a badass like him. He had all these speed records. I wanted my own.

That second night, I passed a group from AmeriCorps doing trail work. I was really exhausted and in a lot of pain. I'd been going since 6 a.m. It was 11 p.m. I sat down next to two young girls and asked how they were doing.

"Do you do this every summer?" I asked.

"Oh, no," one answered. "This is our first time out in the woods. This is the first time we've ever spent any time out in the wilderness. We've never even camped out before this summer."

What? Are you kidding me? They'd been out there a month.

"You've never spent any time out in the wilderness?" I asked.

"Nope," they answered.

I was flabbergasted. I remembered all those times that I acted like a scared little girl in the woods because I was alone, and I was afraid of creatures lurking in the woods. These girls were way younger than me, close to half my age, and they were out there, among the bears, camping out like it was nothing.

They were sweet, so they asked questions about me, and I answered, and they were like whoa, that's cool. But I wanted to hear their stories, and I wanted to tell them something.

"You will remember this the rest of your life," I said.

Then I said I was going into my tent to take a nap, and that I'd be gone by 5 a.m., but I would think about them when I was on the trail. They were clearing the wilderness and taking care of it so people like me could enjoy it. Their packs weighed sixty-five pounds, half their body weight, probably. My pack weighed fifteen pounds.

No way could I bitch now.

The next morning, I popped my blisters, cried, and went on my way.

As I was walking up Muir Pass, it was getting dark, and I was alone, as usual, and all the other hikers were hunkered down, waiting for the sun to slip under the mountains so they could sleep. I really wanted to stop and sleep in the hut. I'd be safer, and I'd sleep better, and I could rest.

But I kept going.

I just wanted to sleep, but as I ran down the pass, leaving the hut and its relative comforts behind me, I couldn't find anywhere that would make a good camping spot. My feet screamed in protest, but my body just seemed resigned to the exhaustion at this point. All I wanted to do was collapse and sleep. The silver lining to not seeing anywhere to rest on the way down meant I had to keep going farther, and I couldn't imagine having to hobble those first few painful steps down a hill. That may make me want to quit.

I got to the bottom of the Pass, where there were some actual campsites. I plopped down at one of those and just lay down and went to sleep. I didn't even take off my trail shoes or get out my tent.

Two days later, I woke up excited because I knew I was close to Tuolumne Meadows. I woke up and splashed some water on my face at 5 a.m., and I washed my crotch and my ass and wiped my arms with some wet wipes. I was just filthy. I was running even more every day at this point, only because I'd gotten so used to the unbelievable pain. But I was also more apt to cry over fresh fruit or snacks. I wanted a shower and a bath and my bed. I wanted to quit. I wanted to be off my feet. I knew they were really bad now. But when I wanted to quit, I would think about my parents, and that was a reminder that some people were sick and couldn't do what I was doing.

On my way to the Meadows, a ranger stopped me. This ranger was known on the Trail for pissing hikers off. She would make you pull out all your stuff out of your pack on the trail so she could see your bear canister. That's an awful thing to do to a backpacker because it takes fifteen minutes to get it all back in, but she didn't care. Bears were a big threat out there, and she wanted everyone to be safe.

She asked for my canister.

"Um," I said. "Uh. Look, I'm going to Reds Meadow. I don't sleep anywhere. I carry minimal gear. I have very little food."

The ranger paused.

"There's reasons we tell you to carry a bear canister," she said.

Bears, I thought. But I didn't say it.

Instead, I promised that I would carry one in the future.

Then she looked at me again.

"I heard you were out here," she said to me. "You are doing something amazing. Go get that speed record."

That was a real pick-me-up. All along the trail, people continued to give me other boosts. They cheered for me and yelled for me and gave me thumbs up.

At this point I was very close to where Ammon was stationed, and my time was almost up, and thank goodness, because I needed to get home. My feet were in awful shape. My blisters were hot and painful to touch and almost bursting. I knew how dirty the rest of my body was, and I couldn't imagine how dirty my feet were at that point.

Only as I went on, nothing looked familiar any longer. I couldn't figure out where I was. The JMT is a long trail, but I knew it pretty well by this point. I'd just hiked it a just week ago, after all. But when it looked like I was heading towards some dam, I really started to worry. I was running for a half hour on the trail at this point.

After a few moments, I saw a packer coming in with his mules. I asked him if I was still on the JMT.

"No," he said, surprised that I would even ask. "You missed the junction."

Without another word, I started crying, turned around, and just started running. I was tired of the trail and of the way I smelled and felt. I alternately limped and hiked, ran and hiked, limped and stumbled. I wanted to get over Donahue Pass, my final obstacle before the Tuolumne Meadows and home.

A mule train went by. I had to move off the trail to fix my blisters, and it was the worst pain I'd felt at that point. Every time I poked a blister, it was like I'd lit it with a match, and pus would start gushing out of it. I just wanted to get to the store at the end of the trail, where I'd see Ammon and finally have some company for the first time in almost a week of misery.

I got to the store at 8 p.m., and it was closed, which was a bummer because I just wanted some French fries, but Ammon was there. He was excited to see me, and I was excited to see him, and he was excited for me because his friend, a nineteen-year-old named Albert, and his twelve-year-old son, Austin, both wanted to pace me to the end.

My feet were not working at all at this point. I had to find some sticks. Austin scoured the woods trying to find a couple for me. It was going to take us all night and into the morning in the freezing valley to get back home. I would still make my goal, thanks to all the time I'd built up by pushing so hard during the trip.

Every couple of hours I had to stop to fix my blisters, if "fixed" can actually describe what I was doing. They were such a mess at this point that I wondered if I was in serious trouble. It was freezing cold, and the two pacers—just boys, really—would huddle together and start falling asleep.

Oh, crap. They're not used to this.

Their well-being was the motivation I needed to keep doing well. I knew at this point I had to keep it together for them. I had to keep them going and keep talking to them to keep them awake.

We were on our final hobble into Yosemite, and we were reaching the junction for Half Dome. I hadn't slept now in twenty-four hours. We're starting to run into a lot more people. The two boys were bragging about me along the way, telling everyone what I was doing since the word hadn't reached hikers who were just starting their journeys or who were hanging for the day in Yosemite.

I ran into a woman who was hiking with her husband. The boys told her what I was doing. She said her husband did the trail too.

"How did you do it in twelve days?" she said, flabbergasted.

I had to correct her and tell her I did it going back and forth in twelve days, yo-yo. She turned and yelled to her husband. "Honey," she said. "Why did it take you so long to do the trail? This woman's done it twice, and she did it way faster than you."

It had taken her husband twenty-one days to do the trail. I told her thanks, and we passed a lot of people towards the end, who often expressed amazement. But the time we reached the end, no one was waiting for us. There was no finish line and no cheering.

Nobody gives a rat's ass.

And yet, when I got to the sign that marked the end, I just bawled. What did I just do? I just did something huge. I'd broken the speed record by four days. Nobody knew it yet but I had my speed record. I cried out of happiness and pride, and I cried because I knew that I got the toughness it required from my mother. I still missed her.

I thanked the boys and made it back to Camp 4, where all the climbers were hanging out. I got into my car and lay down. My feet were trashed. Then Dean Potter, one of the world's most famous climbers who made his mark in Yosemite and continued to spend time there, came over to me.

"I heard about what you just did," he said. "You're a badass. Let me go get a bucket of ice-cold water. You just need to put your feet in it."

When I rose my head, other climbers began to cheer. They came over and told me how impressed they were.

"You totally sent that route," one said, using the climbing lingo to tell me how much of a badass I was. The climbers, who were all about the speed records, totally appreciated my accomplishment. That made me feel awesome.

When I got the energy, I washed my feet since they were disgusting. A doctor I saw later told me to soak them in antibacterial cream and Epsom salt. I had to stay off them for a few days and they eventually would heal up.

I will always remember just being in the back of the van, with my feet dangling over the edge, being cheered by some of the best climbers in the world as we drove away.

That was my finish line.

Ammon and I were the perfect couple, at least according to the world of Yosemite and the climbers who lived there. The truth was, we were far from it.

The second honeymoon that resulted from my speed record didn't last long. I knew things were bad; we were living different lives and had different attitudes. We were an extreme couple, but the truth was, I didn't just want fun. I wanted stability. It didn't take long for Ammon to figure that out either. I didn't need to keep hounding him about getting a job and paying some bills and becoming an adult. He could sense it.

Ammon started acting strangely. He didn't seem to want me around, and yet, when I'd go out on runs, he was always asking where I was going or where I was heading or what I was doing.

Soon, whenever I was in Yosemite—our world, our place—with him, he treated me like an intrusion. After one fight, he told me he didn't want me there any longer, and I left while bawling my head off. I couldn't figure out what I was doing wrong.

During one of these trips, I was upset, and I ran into Jen, a good friend of his who climbed. I knew her only through Ammon, but I really need to talk to someone, so I spilled my guts. She stood there and sympathized, telling me things would get better. It made me feel a little better to unload on someone and hear a little reassurance.

When I got back home, I saw that Ammon's computer was on, so I went to turn it off and saw his email was open. I started to scroll through them, and my heart exploded.

I saw dozens of emails exchanged with Jen, telling each other that they were in love and that she wanted him in the camp with her.

I was furious. If there's one thing I can't stand, it's when people lie or cheat.

I forwarded the worst email to his mother and then called her.

"Your son is a fucking asshole," I yelled into the phone, and then hung up.

When I called Ammon, he didn't pick up his cell phone.

It just sort of ended kind of fucked up like that.

I know it seems like there's no way that a marriage could end that way, right? But it did. He avoided my calls for several months. When I left him a message that I was turning off our cell phone so I didn't have to pay that bill any longer, he texted me to tell me to wait until he got a new one.

He told me that he felt trapped and that he just wanted to do what he wanted to do. He wanted to be a kid, essentially. He never wanted to grow up.

It left me with this open wound in my heart. I had no closure. I felt empty. He made me feel like I wasn't good enough or pretty enough or wild enough. Even though I had known deep down that my relationship with Ammon wasn't going to last, it was the best relationship I'd had up until then. He treated me well for a long time, and he was kind, thoughtful, and encouraging. He had a lot of problems, but he was loving, even if he saw me as some sort of game plan, the way he did with all those other girls.

But Jen fit him better. She smoked pot, drank, and climbed, and she didn't expect him to get a job and pay bills and live a normal life, the way I did. She let him be a kid.

When he did call me, it wasn't to talk. He was usually drunk, and he would say sloppily that he wanted to get back together. Every time he did, it would put another crack in a heart I was trying to mend.

Ironically, when Ammon left, I started to crave his spontaneous side. I wanted someone crazy like him. I wanted someone fun, and I was always looking. I wanted someone outgoing and spontaneous and a kick in the pants, but without the drugs and alcohol.

Although I found out about him and Jen in 2004, our divorce didn't become final until 2006. It took us that long to make it final because he didn't want to talk. My attorney, of course, handled all the paperwork.

Unfortunately, it's hard to find someone intense like me who isn't also a heavy drinker or smoker. It's hard to find someone to date, and it's especially hard when you want someone to be your former lover.

I searched for ways to help myself get over him. I ran a lot, of course, and even though many of the guys I dated were other ultrarunners, they all said, to that man, that I ran too much.

But I wasn't going to stop running. Running was how I got over stuff. It got me through drugs, my father's death, my mother's death, and Suzanne's passing. Running got my endorphins going the way drugs once did; it got me feeling good about myself so I didn't need the drugs any longer. Running helped me through the pain of losing my friends and my family, because when I ran, I was with them. Many times I pretended that I would see them at the finish. They inspired me to run more, to run farther and harder. Running helped keep me sane, but after a while, it was obvious that I would need something else too. I decided to attend a massage school outside of Yosemite.

I used some of the money my mother left me, and I began a three-week course. The idea wasn't to become a massage therapist, since I had no intention of being a massage therapist. I wouldn't leave knowing how to heal others through massage. The idea was to heal myself.

Those three weeks were a true healing experience. Every day, all the attendees would gather in a circle, and the therapist, a Native American, would pass a feather around; when we had the feather, we would talk about things that hurt us in the past. It was very much like a group therapy session.

I emerged from that class ready to try to put myself back to together. And I knew that I would do it back on the trail. Only this time, I wouldn't do it through running.

I would hike the Pacific Crest Trail. All 2,600 miles of it.

Chapter Seventeen

Cursing and Coasting on the Pacific Crest

I first heard about the Pacific Crest Trail (PCT) back in 2000 when I was at the Western States training camp. The trail is the ultimate ultramarathon, a 2,600-mile journey into the Sierra Nevada and Cascade Mountains ranges through California, Oregon, Washington, and Canada. It is a legendary path in my home state of California. If you could complete all of it, people would think you were some kind of legend.

It sounded like a wonderful accomplishment, but it also sounded out of my reach at the time. (This was about the time I was going to take my first multiday backpacking trip with Suzanne and Linda on that Tahoe Rim Trail.)

Part of being an ultrarunner means allowing ideas to bounce around your head until they turn into a dream. When you surround yourself with people who do amazing things, crazy ideas like hiking the whole PCT are actively encouraged, not dismissed. That's honestly how many people enter their first hundred-miler. Others tell them they could do it until they believe it.

And so the idea of hiking the PCT bounced around my head, and I would be reminded of it a few times a year. One of these instances was when I was on the Tahoe Rim, in 2001, and my group ran into two guys who were wearing these huge, monster packs. The three of us stopped to ask them where they were going, to which they responded "Canada."

"Oh my God, you're PCT hikers," I said. "I've never met someone doing that before." I was starstruck and wanted to join them. But I wasn't ready yet. I needed to learn how to backpack and how to grind out twenty-milers on the trail every day. Most of all, I needed to learn how to leave that scared little girl behind in the wilderness.

My record-setting JMT trip taught me all that. I was ready. I just needed a push. Ammon gave me that push.

The JMT was essentially an alternate reality. When completing it, you leave all your material things behind and live out of a backpack. Out there, your only job is to put one foot in front of the other, ignore the loneliness and weariness and survive. It's actually harder than it sounds. You're on your own. You have to find water and plan for food drops and carry your tent and the few things you can carry to protect you from the elements. You have to dodge creatures like bears and mountain lions, and the weather was always overhead, ready to pounce, leaving you soaked and shivering, threatening your progress and, as I would find out, your life.

You even developed an alter ego. Other hikers called me Dirt Diva and that's how I introduced myself to them. I would spend days with these people and sleep next to them and trust them with decisions that could mean my life.

In May 2007, I would take my first step on the PCT.

I needed that alternative reality. I needed to be Dirt Diva.

On May 24, my friend Jerry Roninger dropped me at my starting point in Campo on the Mexican border, and I was on my way.

Jerry and I were longtime friends. I met him in 1997 on top of Mission Peak, and two years later, I saw him again at the Ohlone 50K. He lived near the trailhead of Mission, and I would occasionally see him on the trail as I spent more and more time out there training. He was much older than me—he turned seventy-two in 2017—but he was one of those old guys who reminded me of my father.

I decided to move out of the house we owned together in 2009 since we weren't getting along. I talked to Jerry about renting his spare room, and he thought the extra income and having another ultrarunner in the house would be a good idea. I thought it would be temporary, a few months at most, but at this point I'd began to settle in. He was a big help.

After the first day, I could tell that finishing would be harder than I thought. Right away, the trail began to throw challenges at me that would haunt me the entire trip. It was hotter than I thought it would be, and I was low on water by mile twelve. I ran out of water by mile seventeen, and I struggled and slogged along the path, barely able to finish the first twenty-one miles. Jerry once again proved his worth, as he stuck around, even running the car to the next stop to refill my water bottles, but I wouldn't be able to rely on that the rest of the hike. It was an eye-opener. I'd have to be careful from now on.

On Day 2, after a sleepless night, I ran into three guys who just graduated from college who were going on the trail as a last hurrah before they headed out into the real world. The group was huddled under a tarp, as they didn't go out in the day because it was too hot. They went out in the morning and at night. Whatever, I told them, and got them out from under the tent. I convinced them to get going. I'm glad I did.

Later in the day, we saw a border patrolman. "I suggest you stay together in the next twenty miles," he told us. He told us they had a lot of drug runners and people who smuggle others across the Mexican border; it wasn't safe to camp alone.

That scared me, but at least I wasn't alone. I decided to stay with the college guys.

We hiked another eighteen miles, and we would up trying to hitch a ride into a little town along the way so we could all get a hotel room. I was the one trying to stop the cars. I stuck out my thumb, and a woman stopped.

"I've never stopped for a PCT hitchhiker," she said, "but something told me to stop for you."

I sat up front, while the guys sat in the back.

On Day 5, the guys told me that they were wiped out and calling it quits. They tried to keep up with me and my twenty miles a day, but apparently I was killing them. They decided they couldn't do it any longer.

All of a sudden, for the first time on the trail, I was alone.

I was no longer scared of the wilderness, but it still made me nervous. The PCT seemed to be the wildest place I'd ever been, and it also seemed to attract some of the sketchiest people I'd ever come across. As I hiked, I saw a lot of broken-down trailers that looked like meth labs. They were scary to me.

"I'm out here all alone," I told myself. "People could take me, rape me and kill me, and no one would ever know."

I tried to push those thoughts out of my head, and my stop for the night helped: I headed to a trail angel's cabin. Strangers dotted the trail offered up supplies and places to sleep. Their water stops would save me many times. A guy at this cabin had a screened-in area and a fridge open to hikers where you could take anything you wanted. Hikers tended to congregate there for the night and swap stories. There I met a woman from Europe who had run a couple marathons. These gestures, and the people like me who took advantage of them, always helped salve my nerves and my loneliness.

But early the next morning, I had to get going again. There was always the sun, calling for you to get an early start to avoid the worst of its punishing rays.

I lost my favorite shirt on Day 12, the day before I reached Big Bear City. When I discovered it was gone, I bawled like I'd lost a pet. It had been almost two weeks, and I was already an emotional wreck. I'd go days without speaking to someone. I also exchanged my tent for a tarp, which made it easier and lighter to carry, but it also took away my home, a small creature comfort that had helped soothe my frazzled nerves at night.

I camped that night just off the trail, on a flat spot I cleaned out myself, and collapsed at 10 p.m. Sometimes I found myself stuck between campsites and had to improvise, and this was one of those times. I didn't eat anything. I just went to sleep.

The first light of the morning always woke me up, so around 5:30 a.m., I began to stir, gazing through sleepy, sandy eyes at the dirt around me. When I took a closer look, I sat up, immediately awake.

There were fresh mountain lion prints all around my sleeping bag. I packed up all my things in about a minute and bolted.

On Day 13, I was ten miles from Big Bear City. It was hot again, and I was having a hard time following the trail. It's much better marked now than it was back then because there are many more people attempting to hike all of it. I kept having to pull out my map and book, and I was getting really dehydrated. I began to panic a bit. I felt more alone than ever.

And then I looked down and found a quarter.

My mother was with me, I thought to myself, trying to tell me it would be OK. I would find many coins along the trail from then on, and they all seemed to come just when I needed them, at times I felt lost or afraid or parched. My mother, once again, was watching over me.

At Big Bear, a trail angel ran a hostel where you could share a room for $20. I paid $20, and as a bonus—maybe my mother was watching over me here too—I had the room to myself. I took a bath in a huge tub. Sometimes you could go days on the trail without bathing, and all the sweat and sunscreen and dirt turned your skin into a pie crust. It always felt so good to wash all that off. Many times, the weariness seemed to wash off with it. I had hiked almost three hundred miles at this point.

Big Bear is known for containing Big Bear Lake, one of California's resort destinations, and as I left the next morning, the trail took me to the top of an overpass where I could look down on it and saw all the people swimming and water skiing and diving into deep pools. They were having fun, and I was facing another hot day on the trail, where water was scarce in a dry year and the temperature reached 110 degrees. I tried not to feel sorry for myself as I hiked on and the sun began to bake another thin layer of crust on my skin.

Six days later, on Day 18, Jerry contacted me. He was helping me with my blog while I was on the trail. He had a question for me: there's a guy named Andy Kumeda who wanted to meet me on the trail. Was that all right?

Andy was an ultrarunner. He was training for the Grand Slam, which is a series of four iconic hundred-mile races in one summer. He was getting ready to do the first, a hundred in Old Dominion, Virginia.

I'd seen him at a few races before. We said hi to each other. So sure, Andy could come out and hike with me.

Andy worked a 50K that morning, June 10, and then he drove four hours to meet me along Angeles Crest, the location of one of my favorite hundred-milers. He met me near the Islip Saddle on Highway 2. When I got there, he had a card for me that all the other runners signed for me at the 50K, and he had fresh fruit and even homemade lemonade set up in the back of his vehicle.

The visit really lifted my spirits. Most of the time on the trail you're thinking inside yourself, especially because at times you won't see someone for up to a week. I was thinking about my mom's passing and where my life was heading after the divorce, and though I told myself I was hiking to get over Ammon, I inevitably thought about him a lot, too, and what went wrong. Just knowing that I was going to get a chance to get out of my own head for a bit kept me bouncing along the trail, and that short visit put another hop in my step as I went on. I needed it.

He would stay with me as a result. There was a spark there. Maybe I'd get a chance to explore it.

The days melted into one another after that for a while. I'd usually knock off twenty miles or so a day, and the one constant was my never-ending search for water. The dry year seemed to have sopped up every stream and watering hole where I could get fresh water. This made it difficult, as the books and maps would lead me to a known stream, only to be greeted by sunbaked ground when I got there. There were many days that I barely had enough water to get through another hot day. If it wasn't for the trail angels who left jugs full of water at certain checkpoints, I wouldn't have been able to continue.

This lack of water would start to catch up to me on Day 39, when I began peeing blood after making it through a tough stretch through the Sierras. Yep. You guessed it. Another bladder infection had started to haunt me. The bladder pain began to sharpen around Day 42, when I was forty miles from the Muir Trail Ranch, as by this point the PCT overlapped the JMT. I was moving more slowly than I wanted to because the pain was so bad, and so I ran out of food before my next resupply at the Ranch. I asked a ranger if he had any supplies he could donate to me, and he gave me some stale nuts and rice cakes that he found in one of the bear boxes at a campsite. This was great because the food fit my vegan diet, but they were disgusting.

I made it to the Ranch on Day 44, and the pain felt like a red hot poker in my bladder. It was the worst infection I'd ever had, and I'd had many by now. A doctor said she'd had an infection like mine once and got a prescription after just a few hours. She couldn't believe I went five days with it. She told me to take the medicine and rest for a couple days.

I found a groove again on Day 54, when I hiked thirty-four miles and felt good enough to think about all my nearby ultrarunning friends and how cool it would be to run a fifty-mile race scheduled for nearby Sierra City in Nevada. I had hiked twelve hundred miles by then, and I hadn't run more than a few miles at a time in more than two months. But it also sounded really fun to step back into my circle for a day.

I called Jerry and asked him to bring Rocky, my wiener dog at the time, and when I arrived that morning, I about squeezed the life out of him and basked in all the people who were calling my name and asking me about my adventure. I soaked all of it in, knowing that I would want to remember it later.

I felt great during the race, and I had fun running it and even more fun cheering everyone else on. It felt great to be with my community again. But it made it so much harder to leave two days later.

Jerry and Rocky tagged along beside me for the first two-hundred yards in the morning, and I began to tear up. I started to huff up a big climb, turned back to Jerry and told him to take Rocky and leave. I just couldn't take it any longer.

Jerry said goodbye and Rocky gave me a kiss on the nose, and I began to bawl. I continued crying, hard, the whole way up the hill.

That night it was really cold and windy, and the tears stung against my face. I crawled into my tent and bawled yet again. I felt so alone.

I had grown used to being alone, with an occasional companion to help ease it, but being around people and Rocky again made the solitude stand out. I missed my dog. I missed my old life. I missed my parents.

I missed Ammon.

By Day 77, I was up to seven bear sightings, one bobcat, four foxes, three coyotes, at least a dozen deer, and hundreds of lizards. I had hiked 1,571 miles. I was more than halfway done. This was now the most physically and mentally challenging thing I had done, but a pick-me-up was coming: I was just a few days from Ashland, Oregon, where I would get to visit Hal Koerner's running store, Rogue Valley Runners.

I had had a rough stretch a bit back near Etna, where I couldn't find water yet again and had to settle for a nasty pool of sludgy water next to a sheep pasture that I filtered with my bandana and purified with chlorine tablets.

But things were looking up: my lonely stretches were over. I bonded with a couple hikers. One was named Bull, who got his name because he was a big guy, and Eric the Black, because he wore black. I was excited to show him and other hikers tagging along with us the running store owned by that year's Western States champion in Ashland.

But when we got to the store, the news wasn't as uplifting as I had hoped: we heard that a lot of PCT hikers were getting sick. They all had giardia, a parasite that often is the result of drinking out of backcountry streams without disinfecting the water.

By Day 86, we lost Eric the Black to giardia as well. He decided to stay behind in Ashland. We hoped he could catch us in a few days. I'd be hiking with Bull alone for a few days.

His wife, whose trail name was City Girl, proved herself by hiking the first nine hundred miles of the PCT with him. But she dropped out because she was holding up Bull and she had a chance to get on the *America's Next Top Model* TV show. Priorities, I guess.

I quickly discovered that Bull was a good companion. He could keep up a fast pace, but he didn't try to compete with you. He was quiet but also talked enough to break up the miles you were doing. He was resourceful too.

Oregon's known for its beautiful forests, and we loved walking under their canopies. That night, we watched the sun set, and the sky turned magenta and red and pink and orange, all the colors of my hair. I started at the sky and thought how lucky I was to be there and how far I'd come, more than 1,750 miles.

But I didn't feel well that day either. I didn't eat much, probably two hundred calories, and just wasn't feeling up to drinking much either.

As I went to bed that night, after the sunset, I had my first bout with diarrhea.

It was a sign of things to come.

My running mentor, Mike Palmer, was hosting his annual 50K, the Psychedelic Climacteric in Berkley in the second week of September. I wanted to hike the race in spirit. When Bull stirred and shivered in the cooler weather, I told him that he'd be doing a 50K that day.

He warned me that the farthest he had gone was twenty-five miles.

"Well, you're doing an ultra today," I told him.

I was still having stomach issues, but I told myself to ignore them for now. I was focused, and I thought the virtual 50K would inspire us.

I was right. Bull did great, and we hiked thirty-three miles in eleven hours and thirty minutes.

We were stoked and celebrated, but not too much, as it began to sprinkle that night.

When we woke up, a thick, almost menacing fog surrounded us, accompanying more light rain.

Even so, the weather didn't worry me too much. This wasn't California currently suffering through a dry year. We were well into Oregon by now, with a climate about as close to a rainforest as the continental US can offer, and so Bull and I left that morning more concerned about the rumbling in my stomach than in the sky. I'd had a couple more bouts with diarrhea that night.

We began making good progress. It felt good to warm up in the cool air, the opposite of the oppressive heat that California had tossed to me. We'd even hoped to reach Crater Lake in time to meet up with a guy named Chris who had hiked the whole PCT with his brother back in the early eighties when he was eighteen, and who had been inspired to get back on the trail again after my reading my blog. That made me feel good, and so of course I wanted to talk to him a bit. . We began to cruise up to Oregon's highest point on the PCT just north of Crater Lake National Park, and I was hiking so fast to stay warm that I left Bull behind.

The wind began to pick up as we approached the highest point on the trail in Oregon, about 7,560 feet, just north of Mount Thielsen, referred to as the Lightning Rod of the Cascades. And we were about to find out how it had earned its nickname.

It began pouring, and kept getting colder and windier by the minute. I had a rain jacket, but it was soaked through in no time. I couldn't see Bull at all through the fog, but I decided to keep going to try to stay warm.

It didn't work. The water soaked my gloves to the skin. The rain was relentless.

We'd been hiking for just an hour, and we were in serious trouble. I had to find Bull.

I walked back on the trail, unable to see but hoping to run into him, and I finally saw the faint outline of a guy wrapped in some sort of tarp.

It was Bull. He didn't have much rain protection, so he had wrapped himself in his tent and was stumbling along the trail.

It began to hail, and I got in Bull's face and told him we couldn't go on.

Our hands were frozen, so it was like trying to set up a tent while holding a large rock in each hand. But we managed to pound his stakes into the ground with our stone fists, and we crawled inside, stripped off all our wet clothing and tried to find something dry in our packs. Bull had a stove, and he made tea, and that was a fucking godsend.

We rode out the storm for the next twenty-four hours, freezing, in our sleeping bags, spooned next to one another to try to manufacture any kind of heat. We were shivering and surviving but just barely.

Even now, I always pack warm gear whenever I go for a hike or a long run. I don't ever want to be as cold as I was that night ever again.

The next morning, the weather was better. We crawled out of our tents, shook off the rain and continued on to Crater Lake. It was huge and beautiful and glorious. We met Chris again (who strangely did not have a trail name), and we met back up with Eric the Black.

Things, it seemed, were looking up, but I was unknowingly near the end.

I got up the next morning and looked at myself in the mirror. I hadn't done that in many days, and I immediately got an ugly flashback to my eating disorder. I looked like I'd been thrown down a prison hole with a few slices of bread and water to get me through the month. My clothes were hanging off me, and bones protruded everywhere. I tried not to look for too long, as I didn't want it to bring back any relapses.

My stomach was really angry at this point, and I wonder if that's why I looked so thin. My body just seemed to keep eliminating anything I put into it. I was having explosive diarrhea pretty much all the time.

I was alone again at this point. Bull and Eric the Black decided to take a spur trail down to Mount Hood, and Chris, after six days, had to go back to his real life. I was in my own head again. Maybe that's why I wasn't paying attention to where I was walking.

I stepped on a slick rock, and I slipped. The weight of my heavy pack threw me to the side, and I twisted my knee.

I tried to tough it out. I'd built my reputation as someone who could tough it out. But I couldn't tough this out. I stopped in the next town and went to a clinic.

The doctor confirmed my fears. I had giardia. I'm still not sure where I got it, but I'm assuming drinking out of a fetid pool next to a sheep pasture was probably not the smartest thing to do, no matter how thirsty I was.

She gave me an antibiotic, but with the caveat that that it would made me sicker before it made me better. She looked over my knee, gave me a sympathetic look, and told me that between the giardia and my knee I would need to rest for a couple weeks before things were better.

I considered going on because that's what I do, but ultimately I was still an ultrarunner, and I didn't want to cause any permanent damage that would prevent me from doing more epic things.

On Day 99, in a small motel room in Sisters, Oregon, my journey ended.

I cried for a while. I considered completing the PCT somewhat of a dream, and now it seemed to be over. I felt like such a fucking failure.

So many people had supported me. So many of my friends such as Andy came out to lift my spirits or hike with me, and I felt like I was letting them down, as well as all the trail buddies who traveled with me along the way. My roommate, Jerry, met me many times along the trail to give me some (much-needed) water and supplies. The trip would not have been possible, or nearly as much fun, without all their help.

When I got to the airport, I felt as if I was tossed back into civilization. I was in this busy area and all these things were happening. People were everywhere. I had to stuff myself into an airplane with dozens of other people, drive a packed freeway, and then, suddenly, I was home, with angry bowels, a swollen knee, and a sour attitude.

I couldn't wait to get back on the trail and finish. But during my recovery, my bowels improved, and my knee improved, but the weather that almost killed me and Bull didn't improve. A huge snow storm swept through Washington, clogging the trail full of snow. I contacted Bull to see how bad it was, and he told me not to bother coming out. They were sending search parties out for hikers who were trapped in the snow for more than three days.

I would not complete my main goal for that year.

But I did accomplish one really important goal: I got over Ammon. I'd left him out there, on the trail, where I thought he'd be happier anyway.

As women, we think we're the ones at fault. I'd finally realized that it wasn't my fault and that it was going to be okay. I had healed from that relationship, or at the very least, I was well on my way towards healing.

The trip served its purpose. All the pain and solitude and miles and miles and miles of hiking was worth it.

I could have done without the diarrhea though.

Seven years later, in 2014, at the Wasatch 100 in Utah, Ammon crewed me. We found each other on Facebook, and we began talking again, and after a bit, he said he would come out and act as my crew. I remembered him for his loving nature and his thoughtfulness, and that extended into him being one of the best crew members I'd ever had. So I said yes.

After the race, he told me he regretted how everything worked out. He apologized for it. I got closure. That was something I had always wanted.

I kissed him. But when I did, eight years after the divorce was final and twelve years after we met, it confirmed what I thought. He was not the type of person I wanted to be in a relationship with any longer. I was grateful I wasn't with him any longer.

I'd become a totally different person. I was immersed into my ultra-running community. It was my life now. And I had more races to run.

Chapter Eighteen

Dodging Death in Two Different Ways

As I was driving out to Yosemite, I was looking forward to sharing Donohue Pass with my mentor, Mike Palmer, and friend, Julia Bramer, for a trip in 2011. Mike, of course, was a running partner who had shared many hundred-mile races with me and therefore had seen me at my worst many times. Julia was also a training partner and a good friend, but she was also important to me for a different reason: she did my hair. At this point in my life, my hair was bright pink, with streaks of orange, purple, and an occasional flash of red. My hair, along with my piercings and tattoos, are more than just about looking good. They are an outward symbol of my identity. They are what help make Catra Corbett. That badass identity, along with my accomplishments, has gotten me followers on social media, shoe deals, and race fees comped. But most of all, these parts of my appearance have helped me be Catra the Ultrarunner.

And by being Catra the Ultrarunner, I've stayed off drugs.

It's a nice trade-off.

So I was really excited to show Mike and Julia the Donohue Pass. Donohue is an eleven-thousand-foot pass on the boundary between

Yosemite and Ansel Adams Wilderness. It is the sixth-highest pass of the ten named passes on the John Muir Trail. Because neither of them had even been before, I wanted to share it with them.

Although there had been clear skies that morning, as we were getting our gear together, I made sure that we all brought rain shells. You never know what can happen. Mike knew this all too well too, having been caught in rainstorms with me, including the epic one a few years ago where we almost got struck by lightning.

Once we got out there, it looked amazing, and though I wanted to make sure we got to the top of Donohue Peak by noon, we were taking photos, and I took off ahead the last few miles.

The sky looked clear, or it seemed clear, all the way to the top of the pass.

And then I see these clouds coming off the top of the peak. Not good.

I never knew my sister Peggy very well. When she was a teenager, I was only eight. I remember, growing up, that I would hear things about her. She was the reason I first heard the word "overdose."

My parents would discuss her around me. Peggy was bipolar, but unfortunately, at the time, that wasn't a widespread diagnosis. The doctors didn't know how to treat it. Peggy wound up treating herself by "self-medicating."

We lived in the suburbs but rented a ranch where we had horses, bulls, and steers and Charlie. Peggy was already doing the hard drugs to make herself feel better. And at one point, she started using the horse tranquilizers. She must have been miserable.

As I got older and became a teenager, I wanted her to buy alcohol for me and my friends. Sometimes she would. She was just twenty-one and didn't care. Drugs were the most important thing in her life, which is why her personal life was a wreck.

She got married when she was nineteen, but her husband was a really nice guy, and because of that, she straightened up for a while. She had a house and a kid, and ultimately had a nice life. I loved to go over to her house and hang out with my niece.

A couple years later though, Peggy met up with an old boyfriend. She started cheating on her husband and then left him. It only got worse: Peggy got pregnant by her boyfriend, and then her boyfriend died in an accident, propelling her into hitting heavy drugs, including heroin.

Peggy's kids were passed around between family members. Her son, Joshua, stayed with my mom for a while, and his life was really heartbreaking. On every one of his birthdays and on Christmas, Peggy would call my mother's and tell Joshua that she was coming over with presents, and she wouldn't show. It was constant. The only time she would come around was when she wanted money for drugs.

My mother wanted to save her and wanted to enlist my help. Peggy was still her child, so she would let Peggy live with her when she came back and promised to get clean. She wanted to believe her so badly that she did.

My mother would sometimes believe she had control over her, but of course, she didn't.

The only thing that had control over Peggy was heroin.

It started to get cold by the time I got to the top of the Donohue Pass. I took a few pictures as Mike and Julia approached, and I could see more and more clouds approaching. I heard the first clap of thunder way in the distance.

We gotta go, I thought.

The clouds started covering me.

It started to sprinkle, and the thunder was no longer in the distance.

"We gotta go," I yelled down, and I sprinted back with Mike and Julia.

The storm caught up to us a lot faster than we anticipated. Storms are like that in the mountains. They can literally sneak up on you, forming in minutes, even out of the beauty of a blue sky.

It started to sprinkle, and then it started raining, and then I felt the first bump of ice against my skin, as if someone had thrown a frozen marble at me.

With that, I attempted to take cover under larger trees, but I had to settle for a small grouping of pine trees as Mike and Julia approached from behind. As I waited, the bumps became thumps, and the hail bounced off my flesh. It hurt. I cowered in the group of trees since it was hailing really hard now. It was dangerous.

I began to shiver.

But still, as fast as the storms come, that's also as fast as they usually dissipate. *This should be over in a half hour*, I thought, because that's almost always how storms disappear. *The sun will come out and melt the hail, and I will be warm again.*

Mike, Julia, and I greeted each other at the trees where two hikers, an English couple, had also taken refuge, and Julia looked even worse than I did. The wind began blowing even harder, and the thunder was ringing through our ears. The hail looked like snow at this point. Julia was shaking hard, and we were all freezing, and I realized as the wind tried to blow us over that we are all just soaked through our rain jackets.

This storm had already lasted a half hour, and then an hour, and it didn't seem like it was going to let up soon at all.

I felt terrible for my friends. I had brought them up here. This was supposed to be a day of sharing memories with two good friends. But now we were making nothing but bad memories. Julia was scared, which terrified me. It made me realize that we were in serious trouble.

Things got pretty bad with Peggy after I moved out of the house. My mom would fill me in on her while I was doing her hair. Peggy had resorted to prostitution to pay for her drugs.

Occasionally, my mother would drive around the neighborhood with a friend and go look for her on the streets, then bring her back, show her the kids, and try to work some sense into her. She spent thousands of dollars to put Peggy into rehab.

One time, it seemed to work. Mom paid thirty-thousand dollars for a clinic, and Peggy got straight for six months. She was doing really well, actually gaining weight and looking healthy. But then she got back on again.

Addicts lie a lot; mostly, they lie to themselves about their own condition. Addicts tell themselves that things aren't as bad as they seem. But they are and often they are worse. And watching Peggy go through such a hellish life made it easy for me to lie to myself.

Peggy made it very easy for me to convince myself that I was not a drug addict. I'd tell myself, *Look at Peggy. That is a drug addict.*

When she did visit our house, when I was living with my mom in the early days of my recovery, Peggy would come over and ask about me. She wondered how I could recover. She also wondered why she couldn't if I could.

I told her I found something I loved that helped me forget about the drugs.

"I'm proud of you," Peggy said right away.

Peggy didn't necessarily want to be on drugs. She knew what they were doing to her and saw how they ruined her life. But she also didn't want to give them up, even after she lost everything, including her family, because of them.

She also knew how hard they were to kick. I think she was glad her younger sister was able to kick the drugs. She once cared about me a lot, and I think she was glad that someone like me whom she still loved somewhere in her heart had not only saved her own life but turned it around.

After my mother died, Peggy was in and out of jail. This was the start of her real downfall, and her kids began to disappear as a result.

Joshua was living with his grandmother on his father's side full time. Peggy's eldest child, Vanessa, went to live with her father. Once my mother found out Peggy was really getting bad, she called Vanessa's father and got him full custody. Peggy's two youngest kids were adopted out almost as soon as they were born. This made us very sad.

Even so, Peggy still wanted a place in our family, at least for the money we could give her. When she was released from prison, she came by the house, looking for her share of our mom's estate.

She thought she was going to get a bunch of money from my mother. But my mother was very clear. She left Peggy money, but Peggy wasn't going to get it until she was clean and sober. We could even use the money to get her clean. But she couldn't truly have any of it until she was better.

That pissed Peggy off. "You guys are ripping me off," she would tell Patty and me, and eventually Patty told her she was not welcome in the house any longer.

I never got to talk to her again.

The storm had us trapped. The lightning crashed around us, and the hail wouldn't let us move, pelting us with frozen rocks every time we poked our heads out to contemplate a break for it.

I asked the three guys if they could let us borrow their tarp for their tent and if we could all huddle together. We wrapped ourselves up with complete strangers; it seemed to help but only a little.

The English couple huddled up with us told us that we could all set up their tent, and we could stay in there until things got better. We would have to leave the safety of the trees, but we decided we couldn't stay up there any longer without risking severe hypothermia. We decided we needed to make a run for it.

We stepped on the trail only to be buried in hail. We couldn't see anything in front of us but used our instincts and followed the faint outline of the path as it wound down the pass. The goal was to get to the other side of the creek and set up the English couple's tent. The real goal was to get warm and into safety.

It was only a half mile to the creek, but it felt good to run even just that little portion. I warmed up just a touch. But my delight was tempered after I saw the creek. The storm had turned it into a raging river. The rocks were covered by the fast-moving water. That's what we would have to cross.

We would have to link arms and make it across.

I went first, followed by Mike and then Julia.

The water stung my legs the second I put them in.

I began pulling our chain of people across the river so we could get out as soon as possible. The water was so cold that it burned. From behind me, I heard Julia freaking out.

She was hysterical, screaming at everyone to let her by so she could get across. As she was pulling and yanking on the people, she slipped and fell headfirst into the water.

The storm was still raging, and Julia was soaked and as cold and crazed as she can could be, trembling like an earthquake. But once we were across, we were safe in the trees. The English couple began to set up the tent, while we started our run.

The three of us were so cold that we were running and running without getting warmer. Julia was leading the way. She continued to run, and at this point, we were chasing her as much as we were running ourselves. Finally we stopped.

"Are you okay?" I asked Julia, but I already know the answer. She was a lot better.

Running saved me once again, and this time, it saved my friends too.

When the two police officers came, in 2004, we knew immediately why they were there.

They weren't there for me. I'd long since been off drugs and ultra-running and had a job. I had a life.

"Do you know Peggy Corbett?" they asked us when I answered the door.

I had been thinking about Peggy the days leading up to this day. It had been two years since I had contact with her. I kind of assumed something had happened to her.

"They found Peggy dead in a hotel room," one officer said, and my heart dropped.

It was not a punch in the gut. My family had been waiting for the news for years now, and I knew, then, why I'd been thinking about her.

Apparently, when she died, she was with a group of drug addicts. They were doing drugs, the rest of the group left to go the store, and when they came back, she was dead.

The police said she had been released from jail a couple days before. I didn't even know she was in jail. But that news didn't surprise us either.

They found several different drugs in her system. It was the last straw. She was not able to survive this last overdose.

I don't think she wanted to survive. She had to know that the amount of drugs in her system would kill her. I truly believe she mixed all those drugs together to end the unending suffering her life had become. Many of her friends were already dead from overdoses. Her kids were gone. She knew we didn't want her around.

She, more than anyone else, would know how much heroin could kill a person.

The officers asked me and Patty to identify the body. My sister didn't want to do it, and I didn't want to remember her like that. We had to ask a cousin to do it.

The cousin said Peggy looked really bad. She looked old. Her hard life had aged her. The drugs had aged her.

I was glad I didn't have to see her like that. At least I can remember her in a better place.

Peggy was not able to find something to save her. Now, when I'm struggling in a race, I add Peggy to my list of departed loved ones that I think about. Especially with her, I think about why she couldn't choose life. I think about the sense of relief I felt when she died because I knew she had nothing in her life.

While all addicts hit rock bottom, I think Peggy hit lows that were worse than death. She gave up her kids, worked as a prostitute, and distanced herself from her family, all for drugs. She died in a shitty hotel room, alone.

I know that that could have been me. At the height of my addiction, I didn't see any way out of my life. I never saw the next day. It scares me now to know that I thought that way, since Peggy thought the same way.

My memories of her make the pain better when I'm running a hundred-miler, or when I face a precarious situation because of the adventures I now enjoy.

I was lucky. I found something to love.

Chapter Nineteen

My Wiener-Sized Companions

When I was in the second grade, I, like a lot of other little kids, asked my parents for a dog. My friends were giving away a poodle. I begged. I pleaded. I yearned. They finally gave in.

I named her Candy. She was a great little dog, until she bit me. I was afraid of her after that.

Our neighbors had a German Shepherd. One day when I was passing by their house, the German Shepherd ran out, lunged at me, and nipped me. He didn't hurt me, but that made my fear of dogs much worse. I had a strong foundation of fear of pooches, and the dog didn't help. He was a big dog, and his bark was even bigger, a deep-throated explosion of canine curses. At least it sounded that way to me. He was actually a sweet dog, but by then, I was afraid of any dog, let alone one that made my stomach shake every time he barked. Every time he came over, I would start crying.

We didn't have dogs the rest of my time growing up. Instead, we had cats, which was fine.

When I first met Jason, his parents had this teeny-tiny wiener dog named Twinkie. Twinkie was blind, had cancer, and was in pain most of the time I knew her. She would snap when she sensed someone was close. At this point, I was still afraid of dogs.

"Get her away," I would scream when she tried to bite. "Get her away."

I knew nothing about the breed up until then, but that was my introduction to wiener dogs.

It was the start of an unlikely love affair.

Jason's family called themselves a "wiener dog family." They'd had a pet of that breed for as long as they had been a family.

Twinkie eventually got really sick and needed to be put to sleep. Jason's parents asked me and him to bring her into the vet to have her put down. They just didn't have the heart to do it.

She was still snappy but had missing teeth and putrid breath, but on our way to the vet, I felt something for her. This was the end of her life. After we had arrived and filled out all the paperwork, we left her at the vet without staying for her final moments. When we were driving away, I felt horrible. Who would just drop something off to be put down without staying with her? But we were on drugs, too, and that always clouded our empathy and judgment.

Twinkie stayed on my mind. Soon after, Jason's family got another dachshund, Deedee. I was no longer afraid.

On many days when I wasn't at work, it was just Deedee and me in the house. We spent so much time together that I fell in love with her. She was my sole true companion during that dark time.

When Jason and I broke up and I left the house, Deedee was the only piece of my old life I held onto. I had an agreement with Jason that I could have her every weekend. Eventually, Jason asked if I wanted my own wiener dog, and offered to pay for half of it. I immediately agreed.

We went to the dachshund breeder soon after, and as I looked in a pile of squirming puppies, I saw one of them seemed completely out of control. He was running around, crashing into his siblings, and jumping everywhere. He looked as if someone had wound him up and broken off the key so he would stay that way forever.

"I want that one," I told the attendant. I named him Oskar, as in "Oscar Meyer wiener."

Oskar really was crazy, but I loved him. He was my first wiener dog, my little love bug, my first running partner. Plus, he went through my recovery with me.

I tried taking him on my first few runs, and he got up to six miles, which was a big accomplishment for both him and me. I was living with my mom at the time, and Oskar bonded with her, too, especially on the four-mile walks that she frequently took to get herself in better shape.

When my running took off, and as I got into marathons and then ultras, Oskar slowed down. And he got older.

Soon after my mother died, Oskar went too. I was really upset, but Oskar did his job. He made me realize I could keep a dog of my own and love it and rely on it for companionship. I would need those dogs in my life even more than I initially thought.

After Oskar died, Mike, my mentor, would send me emails of dogs up for adoption. I wasn't ready to get another one yet; that is, I wasn't ready until I opened an email and saw Rocky near the end of 2003.

It had been a year, and I missed Oskar. I missed that companionship.

Rocky looked like a dachshund mixed with some other breed. He was really cute. A woman who ran a foster adoption center for small breed dogs had found him wandering the streets. I agreed to drive there to take a look at him.

Mike and I drove up to a house in shambles.

"Come around the back," we heard a woman called out.

We waded through weeds, dog poop, and piles of trash to a trailer in the backyard. The woman opened the door and all these yapping little dogs burst out barking. One of them was Rocky.

Mike went down to pet him and Rocky bit him.

"He doesn't like men," the woman said.

When I bent down, Rocky came up to me, and the woman seemed surprised. "He likes you," she said. I liked him too and so I decided to adopt him.

I paid the necessary adoption and immunization fees, and the woman said she would need to have him fixed first before I could take him. She told me that I would hear from her soon, and I left that day excited for my new canine companion.

Mike picked up Rocky once he was ready, and Rocky loved Mike after that. I think it's because Mike was the one who took him away from that place. Mike rescued him. Every time Mike came over to the house, Rocky would do this crazy little dance of happiness.

I started Rocky running with me soon after I brought him home. I found out quickly that Rocky, like me, didn't seem to like running on the road much. But when I took him out to a trail, he really seemed to enjoy it. The trail was quiet and he could be free there.

Rocky was a smart dog who never left my side, and though he never ran farther than a half marathon, he loved to go out running. His tongue would hang out, and he would just jump and jump, like a jackrabbit. He was a confident, outgoing dog who thought he was much bigger than he was. Whenever he saw big dogs, he would challenge them.

We became very close. A year after I got him, when Ammon and I began having a lot of issues, Rocky was there for me. He was there when our relationship ended. When I decided to do the Pacific Crest Trail to heal my broken heart, I missed him so much. You miss your friends out in the wilderness, but you miss your dog even more.

As more people began to follow my blog, Rocky began to get his own fans, and one made him his own Facebook page. He was a happy dog and loved all the attention.

Rocky also loved food and was always getting into stuff. He would eat anything, constantly digging into my running gels and other people food. One day, it caught up to him.

He was an older dog. We think he was about eleven years old by this point. But he still didn't seem right, so I took him to the vet. She assumed he had eaten something bad, gave him charcoal to induce vomiting, and sent him home with instructions to keep an eye on him until he threw up. It didn't seem to work. He started whining and was wobbly on his feet. He was drooling and bumping into walls. I took him back to the vet, but she didn't seem super concerned. I left him there overnight, thinking he was going to get better.

The vet called me later in the morning.

"It's not looking good," she said.

My heart shattered.

"Is there anything we can do?" I asked.

"No," she answered. "I'll keep him alive until you get here."

When I got to the vet, I thanked him for the eight years he was with me and I told him how sorry I was that he had to go. And then I watched him leave this earth.

I thought about how happy he would be to be able to visit Oskar and my mom, and perhaps to meet my dad. It helped to think about him with them, but it left me absolutely devastated. I needed him. I didn't think I would ever feel better.

Almost every ultrarunner I knew sent me cards and flowers after Rocky's passing. I could tell they were all sad to see him go too. He would give everyone a little bit of energy before those races, and in ultramarathons, energy is a precious thing.

I would need help to get over his death. But Rocky did leave for a reason. Had he not left me, I never would have rescued TruMan.

I didn't want another dog for a while after Rocky, but I missed having a dog. I missed having a constant running partner. I missed all the little habits that you form with your pet. But I couldn't take on another dog yet. I couldn't take the pain of losing another one.

My roommate, Jerry, worked at the animal shelter. Animal shelters do amazing things, but they are sad places. But there are volunteers who take the animals out for some playtime, and there are a few others who agree to foster them so the animals can live in a home that will love them and prepare them for adoption.

Jerry suggested that we foster a dog. We would be doing a good service, and even better, get some of the benefits of owning a dog without the heartbreak of losing one. We both missed Rocky. I agreed to do it.

Two days later, a rescue volunteer brought over a little red wiener. She was found wandering the streets, just like Rocky. He called her Skye.

Skye was outgoing and friendly. She was the first of a half-dozen doxies that we fostered. I loved taking them out and running with them and playing with them and figuring out their personalities. I helped to socialize them and get them ready for their permanent homes. They were all super cute and were all loving, nice dogs. I was feeling pretty good about being a foster mom. I'd been a good foster mom for four months, and I'd helped three dogs find forever homes. And then TruMan came into my life.

One day, in August of 2012, Jerry called me during a run in Yosemite.

"We got a foster," he said, "and he's super scared of everything. When you get home, he'll probably be hiding behind a chair."

Great.

It was true that my little boost of affection helped all those dogs get adopted, but they also helped themselves. All the dogs we had fostered were often cute, super-outgoing little creatures who loved attention and loved people. When I walked in the house that day, excited and ready to take on this latest challenge, I knew we weren't getting an easy dog like the previous ones.

It was quiet and I called for him, but he didn't pop out. I looked around the chair, and I saw him in a corner, balled up like a dust bunny. *How sad*, I thought. I didn't want to pull him out of there. I decided to let him come to me. I decided to wait.

I sat there watching him, and after about thirty minutes passed, he poked his head out. He saw me watching and immediately poked his head back in.

Soon after, he stuck his head back out again, and I decided to pull him out of there after all. He was a little timid, but I got the sense he would be alright with me.

He didn't growl, snap, or whine as I dragged him out. He just shook. I sat him on my lap, and he looked at me with his tail tucked under his legs, his ears down, and his body trembling.

"Why are you like this?" I asked him.

I learned that TruMan came from a hoarding house. The woman who owned the house meant well, but she had twenty-one other dogs. With that many dogs, more dominant ones formed a pack and a pecking order. TruMan was at the bottom, and he hid so he wouldn't have to face abuse from the other dogs. At one point, he was adopted out to another woman who worked at a vet hospital who didn't realize how frightened he was. She gave him back, since she thought he was always going to be kind of broken.

Let's just see about that, I thought.

I wasn't ready to adopt another dog, but I was fine taking on a project. It was going to be a lot of work to get him adoptable.

The first day didn't go well. I brought TruMan outside for a walk, and he froze, digging in his heels. He shook when a car passed him by. This dog also didn't seem to like the wildness of the city after living such a chaotic life. The cars and their noise, uncertainty, and size scared him.

So I decided to take him where I went to fix myself after I'd been broken more than once. I took him out front. I went to my old standby trail, Mission Peak, where I'd hiked and ran more than a thousand times by this point. There were no cars—just the dirt, other hikers, and my footfalls.

I sat him on the ground. I wanted to see if this broken dog could mend himself the way I had. I knew there was a good chance he would stay still, but I started running anyway.

He started following me.

I kept running, and he kept following me. His tongue slipped out of his mouth, and he began to bounce a bit. He seemed to enjoy it. The trails seemed to work for him.

It was a start.

The next morning, we went to the trail again. I sat out on the ground, with the dog in my lap. Cars swooshed by, and TruMan squeezed behind me, trembling.

As the cars went by, he shook a little less, and then he stopped.

After a while, I felt his body relax. He came out and sat in my lap again and looked out on the street where all those scary, noisy metal things were zooming by. He was scared, but he wasn't terrified.

Soon after, I took him out on a leash, and I had to drag him for a bit at first. But then he remembered that he wasn't in danger and began to walk by my side.

I began to see him coming around and began to think that he was ready to be put up for adoption. *He would be really good for an elderly lady*, I thought, *someone who wouldn't mind him sitting in her lap all day.*

But after a few weeks, I began to reconsider.

This poor dog had lived in a house for years balled up behind a couch. I got him out of his shell and on the trail. Did I want to put him back there again? Did I want him to live indoors the rest of his life?

No. I was going to make him mine. We are going to be great partners. I wanted him to experience the world. So I saw it as my duty to show him the world.

I adopted him.

TruMan and I would normally run around eight miles together, but on the weekends, I would take him on a longer run and stretch the distance, just like I would for myself. I took him to Yosemite and showed him the different formations out there. I showed him Half Dome, the mountain I kept on my wall, and El Capitan, the mountain where many of my friends climbed and where my ex-husband made his reputation. I took him up mountains, where people cheered for him when he made the top, and I kept running him and waited for him to get tired.

Only TruMan never really got tired. I took him on a ten-mile run, and then twelve, and then we did his first half marathon, and then, in 2014, he did his first full marathon. By 2015, on a boiling hot day in August, he became the first doxen to run a 50K. Three years after I got him, he left that broken dog self behind and became an ultrarunning wiener dog.

I've heard from many people that you shouldn't run a wiener dog because that would cause them to develop leg, hip, and back problems. Disbelievers told me that I was damaging him. They told me I was breaking him. So giving into pressure, I finally took him to the vet, and I got him a full-body X-ray just to see if what people were saying was true.

The vet took a close look at his body and examined him for arthritis in his spine, legs, or hips. The vet came back smiling.

"He's in excellent shape," he said. "He's just amazing."

And he truly is.

TruMan is living a life he never would have had otherwise had he not been in my company. If I wasn't his human, it's possible that his full potential would have never been harnessed.

He's living the life he's supposed to live. When I put a bib on him, he knows what it means. His tongue slips out of his mouth, his ears flop around, and he begins to run behind me. He follows me, usually all the way to the finish.

He is my pacer. He is my dog.

I saved him, and in many ways, he saved me too.

Chapter Twenty

A Hundred Miles, a Hundred Times

Many people would probably call my running an addiction.

I can't blame them. At times, I have thought of it that way myself. In a brief stretch of time, I'd run sixty hundred-mile races, as well as many other ultramarathons. There were times when I raced every weekend. I ran through blisters, bladder infections, and many bad days.

The thing is, running isn't an addiction in the same way I was addicted to meth. I don't feel trapped in a life of running the way I felt trapped by drugs. I don't have to run. I choose to run. And that choice makes all the difference.

Andy wasn't much more than a guy who just came out to give me some trail-angel love on the PCT and save me from freaking out. I thought he was sweet, and he lingered in my head for miles on the PCT, but we said our good-byes. We emailed occasionally after that, but we didn't see each other again until many months later at the Hurt 100.

The Hurt 100 is one of my favorite ultramarathons. Held in Hawaii, it is one of the hardest hundreds in the world. The race itself was uneventful, but after the race, Andy gave me a ride back to my niece's house, and we hung out after the race and talked all night. Eventually we kissed. We spent time together at the airport the next day and made arrangements for me to come down to SoCal for his birthday in January.

I was excited. Andy, for one, was a real ultramarathoner, a shared interest that I'd never had in any other serious relationship before. It would be great to talk about running with someone who was committed to it as much as I was, and who understood why I run hundred-milers.

But beyond that, Andy was a cool guy. He was a mellow, comfortable person to be around. I was still looking for a replacement for Ammon. I had been dating guys in a long search for someone as passionate as Ammon, and as a result, I dealt with a lot of fucked-up guys. Andy, to put it simply, was nothing like those other guys. I was finally ready for a good, healthy relationship. There was a connection there, and we officially began dating after his birthday.

Andy lived several hours away from me, and while I wasn't looking for a long-distance relationship, we made it work when we could. In June, five months after his birthday, we completed our first hundred together in San Diego.

I was much slower than Andy, but he was sweet and stayed with me the whole way, even though the unspoken rule of running a race with someone was that you speed up or slow down at your own pace, regardless of the other person.

The race was eventful for us. We laughed, cried, and yelled at each other, probably because I was melting down. We did all those wonderful things you do when you're running an ultra. We were a good match and pulled each other long.

We were there to stick it out together, and we finished together. It was awesome to finish a hundred-miler with someone who I considered my partner. I'd never felt that before. It felt great. We went on to run lots of races and have lots of adventures together.

The problem was building a life together beyond those races.

Many times over the course of my relationship with Andy, we talked about me moving to southern California. But it never really seemed to happen.

Dating someone from southern California was a lot of work, and it always felt like I was driving there to see him. I would leave Thursday after work, and I'd get up at 3 a.m. on Monday morning to make it back to work. It was a lot.

Andy was mellow and calm, and while I loved that about him, that also meant he was quiet. He was quiet about what he was feeling and thinking. I didn't love that about him.

I'm a super emotional person. I have meltdowns, I scream, and I cry. Sometimes it seemed like our emotional differences might be too much to overcome.

I used to recommend that Andy go to therapy, but he never did. As I've learned, you can only suggest that people talk to a therapist; they have to decide to go because they want to go.

I felt like Andy was more friend than lover. I didn't feel the passion that I felt for Ammon. Andy, like all the guys I dated after Ammon, simply was not Ammon.

But Andy gave me a lot of things. When Rocky died, it was devastating to both of us, and we helped each other through that. But it also was probably our last thing holding us together.

We eventually broke up over the phone on New Year's Day in 2013. Immaturely, I said a bunch of mean stuff to him.

I was devastated not because I lost a lover, but because I lost a friend. I was with him almost every weekend, and now he was gone.

We had both signed up to do the Hurt 100, where we first got together, that same month, but he decided not to go. I decided to go to try to heal myself and get some closure. It made me realize I could do things without him.

My breakup with Andy made me wonder why my relationships didn't work out. I got divorced from a guy I loved with the kind of passion I'd never felt before, and now I was breaking up with a guy who I considered one of my best friends. I couldn't seem to find a happy medium of the two.

I was going through the motions in life without any real purpose, and I hit a dark spot. I became depressed, almost as depressed as I was when I got off drugs. The worst part about it was running felt stale. I just went out and did it. I didn't really want to do it, but I felt like I had to. If I didn't do it, I'd go crazy, and maybe I'd even get back on drugs.

And with no direction, it was getting harder to get out of bed for a run in the morning. It was getting harder to get out of bed at all.

I would turn to my running even as it continued to feel stale. I had a run streak going. I'd run every day since November 9, 2012, and I wasn't going to let anyone ruin that.

Every day, when I felt that dark grind of depression trying to keep me in bed, I'd look at TruMan looking back up at me, and I'd say to myself, *Well, what are you gonna do*? I wasn't going to keep him indoors because I felt sad. He'd been indoors his whole life. I owed it to myself to stay in shape and keep running, but I owed it to TruMan even more.

I didn't want to keep him from having the awesome life I promised him. TruMan saved me because I wanted a better life for him, and that gave me a better life for me too.

It is not easy to run a hundred miles. *No shit, right?* But it's especially hard to run several in one year.

I ran many in a year. In some years, I ran one a month, and there were periods when I was running those races two or three weeks in a row. From 2004 through 2006, I was living out of my van, basically, since it was a convenient place to stay before my runs. I was living like a dirt-bag climber. There were years I did more than a dozen hundred-milers, even some solo hundred-milers.

It was a lot of work and was taxing mentally as well as physically. In fact, it was so tiring that I became extremely depressed. I was basically running hundreds, and in between those, I was recovering and then tapering. It was just too much.

Running races is a wonderful privilege, and that's why you train, but most runners will tell you they get just as much out of the practice of training as they do out of the game day of racing. There's a certain joy in going out for a simple run up Mission Peak, which I've done more than four thousand times, before I go to work. It starts my day off right,

puts me to sleep at night, and clears my head. But when I was tapering, I couldn't do Mission Peak. I had to settle for a simple, shitty little
run around the neighborhood. I couldn't do any of my favorite trails. I
felt lost without that daily routine. I'm convinced that's what led to my
depression: I had no way to clear my head during the week, and then I
had to race on the weekend. And racing doesn't clear your mind. In fact,
sometimes it does the opposite.

Without a doubt, races can be stressful. There's a lot of planning
involved. You have to travel to the race site, attend the expo, and make
sure you've got all your stuff ready for it. Sometimes, because I am a
sponsored runner with Hoka, I had to speak at the expo.

When you're running a hundred or longer, you need to line up a
crew or check what's being served at the aid stations, and you need to
pack the thousand little things that will help you through the day, and
the night, and the next morning, because you will be running for that
long. And the biggest part is completely out of your hands: you have to
hope that your body allows you to run a hundred miles.

Needless to say, it's a lot.

Frequent ultrarunners develop all kinds of major injuries, but I was
relatively fortunate in that sense. I had some hamstring problems, but
that usually bothered me much more when I was sitting down, or riding
in a car, or on a plane. It never seemed to hurt when I was running.

My physical issues were internal—a bladder that just never seemed
to cooperate. It became a real problem as I was trying to do more than a
few races a year.

I got my first bladder infection in 2002, and since then, I never knew
when I'd get one during a race. They always lurked in the background,
threatening my race: when I developed one, they were always very painful, many times to the point where I couldn't finish. I hated the pain, but
I hated the fact that something I couldn't control would screw me out of
a finish. If I don't finish because I am too tired, or because of an injury,
then that's on me. It means I didn't train hard enough. There was nothing I could do for bladder infections. It wasn't fair.

This really hit home in 2005 when a bladder infection forced me to
drop out of Western States. My cramps hurt so bad that I had to sit in a
stream to calm the sharp pain that had been coursing through my abdomen. They were still so strong a few days after a race that I passed out

getting ready for work, which sent me to the hospital. A doctor referred me to an urologist.

The urologist suggested that I take an antibiotic before racing. This was an eye-opener to me. I'd just learned to deal with bladder infections. I didn't realize that there was something you could take that would prevent them. The urologist prescribed Levaquin, but stupidly, I didn't read up on it. He said he gave it to other athletes, and besides, I was excited at the prospect of actually being able to do something about these infections. They hurt, and they were keeping me from doing all the races I wanted to do. I was ready to try anything. I took it before another hundred-miler soon after Western States.

That day, my joints hurt, which was unusual for me, and I felt very weak. I did 100K instead of a hundred-miler, and by the time I was done, I could hardly walk back to my car. When I did read up on Levaquin after the race, it said that runners shouldn't use it because of an increased risk of tendinitis, which pissed me off. When I confronted the urologist about it, he answered that no one else complained before.

Screw him, I thought.

The problem was, the horrendous infections continued. I found a supplement designed to promote urinary track health, D-Mannose. It comes in a powder form that I could put into water. During a race, when I feel the knife start to slip into my abdomen again, I'd put a packet into water and start drinking; that seemed to clear it up.

That only worked for a while. The bladder infections continued to haunt me, and when I was going for my tenth hundred-miler at the San Diego 100 in 2015, something that no one had ever done, the knife worked its way into me again, and this time the pain was awful. When I stopped at the next aid station, at mile thirty-six, a medic asked to see my urine. It came out as a cup of pure blood.

I thought about shuffling along because I really wanted that tenth finish. But it hurt too much. I was devastated. I wanted to be the first to accomplish that. I was really sick of the infections keeping me from what I loved. Nothing else, from the powder to drinking enough during a race to cranberry juice, was working. I decided to go to the urologist again.

When I returned to him, ten years later, in 2015, he apologized for the antibiotic, and he said he read more on it after my problems and said that I was right, that many athletes had many problems with it. Then he said he had something I could use: nitrofurantoin mono.

I now take it one hour before a hundred-mile race and another twelve hours into it. I haven't had another bad infection while racing since then.

It's been a huge relief not to have the possibility of another infection eating away at me during a race. I know now that I can just relax and focus on enjoying my next hundred-miler.

When Andy and I broke up in 2013, I saw that I had fourteen hundred-milers left before I would reach one hundred hundred-milers, which includes solo hundreds of a hundred miles or more. This would be a significant milestone even in the crazy world of ultrarunning. If I reached that goal, I would be only the second woman in the world to achieve it.

The goal was always in the back of my mind, but it wasn't the reason I was running so many hundred-milers. I did dig being Catra Corbett, the woman known for doing epic shit, and the prestige that came with that, and doing all those hundreds was a big part of that. But mostly I just enjoyed the races and appreciated the purpose they brought to my life.

I began picking them off. It would be a tough 2013, I knew. But it would also be a way for me to assert my independence and work through the severe depression I felt after our breakup.

It was a grind, as I knew it would be, but many of the races went well.

The Razorback Endurance Race in San Martin, California, was close to home for me. It was my fourth race of the year and my second hundred of the year. Two weeks before I had finished a fifty-miler, the San Bruno Ultramarathon, and I moved pretty well in that race. I ran it hard and finished first female. I relished in the speed. I was feeling good.

I had a good start, and I kept feeling good. I may have felt too good. The course was flat, and I wanted to prove to myself that I had it in me to do a fast race.

I am faster than some runners who complete hundred-milers. But the reason I am well-known in the ultrarunning world is for my endurance. There aren't many who can run multiple hundred-milers in a year.

Most runners, even the elite ones, won't do more than two marathons in a year.

I don't run those hundred-milers to win. I run them to finish. It's a different mentality. But in this race, I had speed on my mind. I was tired of being known as a plodder and wanted to cut loose.

I knew I had trained enough that I could run a fast time, and I knew this course—a two-mile loop on a flat course—would allow me to do it.

The night before running the Razorback, I laid everything out on a table because I was without a crew, and I told myself that I would not stop. These two-mile courses are very rare in the ultrarunning world, and they are especially dangerous because you get a chance to rest every two miles if you choose to do so. You can come in and stop to talk and fiddle around, and yet your watch keeps burning through the minutes. The best way to lose your motivation is stopping. I knew that if I wanted to run a fast time, I would have to keep moving for this one. I spread out my supplies so I could grab what I needed and go.

Once the gun went off, I began looping, and right from the start I was feeling good. My energy was fantastic. I knew that that would change, of course, but I wanted to ride it as long as I could.

I completed my first marathon in 4:15. I couldn't believe it. That's a really solid marathon for most runners. My 50K was in 5:15, a PR (personal record) at that distance, and my fifty-miler clocked in at 8:25, which was fifteen minutes faster than my best time.

I couldn't believe how fast I was running and how good I felt. I initially told Jerry, who had come out to pace me, that I would be at the 100K mark in fourteen hours. I passed it in twelve.

You just never know how a race will go until you start a race. I'm usually pretty good about nailing a time for someone to meet me somewhere because I normally don't waver from my standard pace. This race was different. I wasn't talking. I wasn't stopping. I was just pushing, pushing, pushing.

I knew from updates from race officials during the two-mile loops that I was first place female and fourth overall, and I was really good with that. I was pushing really hard for up to seventy-five miles, and at some point, the two guys ahead of me dropped.

And then I passed someone, but I didn't think about what that meant until I then heard from an official that I was leading the race. It sounded like a challenge. A glorious challenge, to be sure, but there was no way I was going to coast or back off now.

My stomach started barking at me around that time, and I was trying to block that out. I thought about my sister, Suzanne, my other dogs who had passed away, and my parents; I thought about all those people who I use as my pacers to propel me forward.

It worked for a bit, but my stomach kept acting up, and so I took a walk break. The break lasted longer than I had hoped it would, and by the time I got to eighty miles, I fell apart.

I had severe diarrhea by then. On one of the two-mile loops, I had to stop three times. It was miserable. My pacer kept me going, telling me funny stories, and I just kept shuffling along the last twenty miles, but I was so, so out of it. My stomach hurt so much until the end, when I crossed the finish line as the winner.

Not too many women ever win a race, let alone a hundred-mile race, and I was thrilled. It was so unlike me, and it felt very fulfilling. I ran twenty-one hours. I cut an hour off my PR. Right after I finished, I had bloody diarrhea and began throwing up. My body just wasn't used to going that hard for that long.

The puke looked like coffee grounds. I wondered if it was because of all the dates I was eating, but the medics told me that meant I was bleeding internally. I went to see a gastrologist, who performed an endoscopy. The results showed that I had an internal sunburn from all the Advil I took. I took nine in twenty-four hours. They gave me some prescription heartburn medication.

This caught up to me in the next race, Western States. I began to dry heave about halfway through the race, and I still had bloody stools and had no energy. Again, when I run what I would call a normal hundred miles, with the realization on how stupid that sounds, I'd proven that I could recover well. But running a race hard takes a lot of recovery time. Even the best marathoners in the world only do a couple elite races a year. That's because they run hard.

At the medic tent, they pulled me at mile eighty-five, which sounds crazy because I was done, until you realize I still had more than a half-marathon to go. They gave me an IV and put a wool blanket over me.

It was the same scratchy, shitty kind of blanket like the one the police gave me when I was in jail. It instantly brought back a lot of horrible memories. In fact, it symbolized the fear I had of prison and why drugs no longer appealed to me anymore. I would think about that blanket as much as I would the other women or the long night behind bars with them.

"GET THIS OFF ME!"

They took it off right away.

My final push toward the hundred-mile goal started with the Javelina Jundred, a 100K or hundred-mile race in the McDowell Mountain Regional Park, just north of Fountain Hills, Arizona. If there was ever a hundred-miler that seemed to be created just for me, this was it.

The race itself is always held close to Halloween—the 2017 race took place the weekend before—and many runners dress up in costumes. This, of course, fits my personality perfectly. I love bright colors because they're exactly the opposite of what I used to wear when I was a Goth and I love pink because pink is positive. It makes me feel good. It helps me stay in my head when I'm struggling.

I always have fun at Javelina. I love to think about my costume for months in advance, and everyone seems to want to know what I'll pick out. That year, in 2013, I was a little neon-colored witch and TruMan had a matching costume. In fact, he had five matching-costumes.

The Javelina Jundred consists of five, twenty-two-mile loops (yes, they cut the last one a bit short) on the Escondido Trail, and I had someone change his outfit for every loop. It was a great time, and I finished it.

I should have be stoked for at Run d'Amore. After all, this was the race that would give me a hundred hundred-milers. I'd become only the fifth person in the world to run that many hundred-milers. A lot of my friends would be there to support me and celebrate with me because it was a close, easier race, at least for a hundred-miler.

It was a time to celebrate all those mundane miles and all the work I'd put into being able to do them. But I didn't want to make it a big to-do.

Ultrarunning is such a selfish sport. You have to sacrifice time with your friends, your lovers, and your dog, even when they're runners, all so you can focus on some weird goal or chasing some achievement. Chasing those achievements was a healthy outlet for me, but in a way, it was also selfish, even without me having children or a husband.

Run d'Amore was like so many other races. It was a looped, basic course. I had no serious issues and finished in twenty-six hours.

I did care a lot during the race. I was crying in the middle of it. I thought of the people who couldn't be there who would be thrilled to see it. I thought my mother would be proud. I thought my father would be amazed. I even thought my sister Peggy would think it was great.

But at the end, I just finished. I was drained from all the racing that year. It was nice to get all the congrats from my friends and move on. No fanfare needed. This felt more like an unfinished accomplishment. It wasn't the end.

By the end of summer 2017, I was up to 131 ultras. These are races and solo runs I've done. I have also run twenty-five solo runs of a hundred miles or more, including my first solo in Yosemite. I also count a few two-hundred-mile races in those.

I may have the most woman finishes for one hundred or more miles. I'm honestly not sure. There aren't many who have done one hundred miles a hundred times.

It doesn't matter. It's my thing. It's something I do for me.

It's something I do to keep me off drugs.

However, it is not an addiction. An addiction, by definition, is an activity that you do despite the severe harm it causes. Ultrarunning is just the opposite of that for me, even with all the pain it causes.

I guess it is an obsession. It gives me something in my life. If I didn't have this, I would have to have something else in my life.

One day, when I can't run, I hope I can still hike, but I hope to run as long as possible. There are still ladies in their seventies doing hundreds.

I hope to be one of them one day.

Chapter Twenty-One

A Run for a Lifetime

In January 2016, I got an email from Charlie Engle asking if I'd be interested in running across the continental US. He was calling it the Icebreaker Run.

Charlie has a story pretty similar to my own. He was a serious addict until 1992. He'd had several close calls as he tried to buy cocaine during his late-night binges. On one of those binges, his car was riddled with bullets in Wichita, Kansas, and that scared him straight. He hasn't used any drugs or alcohol subsequently. Since then he'd done some amazing things, including place fifth in Badwater, a 135-mile race across Death Valley, in 2007 and place fourth in 2009. He won a 250K race in China in 2003. Despite having a reputation as a somewhat acerbic guy, he was also well respected in the ultrarunning community for his accomplishments.

Charlie attempted to run across the country back in 2008 but got injured, and eventually his running partner and fellow Badwater legend, Marshall Ulrich, finished the race in record time without him.

I'd only met Charlie once before, briefly, at the start of a Western States 100 a few years prior, but I was excited about his reason for wanting to do the run. He was running across the country to spread awareness about mental health and drug addiction. He christened it the Icebreaker Run because we were out there to encourage people to start talking about their addictions or their struggle with mental health issues.

"Yes, yes, yes," I said. My sister used drugs to help herself feel better. I struggled with depression and anxiety at times, was a former addict, and almost committed suicide. Even little TruMan had PTSD from his traumatic time with that hoarder lady. We were in.

Our team consisted of David Clark, who was once obese and a drug addict but was now an ultramarathoner who ran the Boston Marathon four years in a row by 2015; Pam Rickard, a former alcoholic who ran several marathons and works for the Herren Project, an organization that helps addicts take the first steps towards recovery; Sophie Kashurba, who struggled with depression and whose mother was an ultrarunner; and Chris Martin, an ultrarunner who struggled with mental health and had the idea to put together the run.

The run would start in Santa Monica, California and span 3,100 miles in twenty-four days, ending in Washington, DC, where Mental Health America was hosting its annual conference. Every runner would have to go five hours a day for more than twenty miles a day.

While I was initially nervous about the trip, I had some advantages. Not everyone on the team had run a hundred miles before, and not everyone was used to that kind of grind. But I was going to be the slowest one, and I didn't want to hold everyone up. I didn't want to be the weak link.

I was also excited to be a part of this historic team. I'd never been a part of any run like this or on any team that was working toward an important goal, one that would potentially help many different people.

I had no idea how it would work. We honestly had no clue how this was going to come together until we all got to Santa Monica in May to run it. Charlie wasn't into communicating beforehand. In fact, it was so disorganized at first that I found out with just a few days warning that I would have to drive to Los Angles from Fremont despite previous plans for me to be picked up.

Once I got to LA, the first thing we collectively figured out was exactly how long we all would be running.

We formed into teams of two. One team shared eight hours of running every day between the two-person team. That meant, essentially, that we were running every sixteen hours. We would be running up to twenty miles a day, or the longest run many do during the peak of their marathon training. It was up to the two-person team to cover the seven hours however they wanted, but generally that meant you were running up to four hours a day.

This made each leg interesting for the runner. You were running at all times of the day and night during the trip, and it didn't seem as if there was a good time to be out there. In the early morning you'd want to be asleep, or during the mid-morning you'd be battling traffic, or in the afternoon, you'd be battling the heat of the day. In the middle of the night, you wanted to be asleep.

When you weren't running, you were riding in an RV all the time, bouncing around. It was close to impossible to sleep like that, so we decided to get hotel rooms.

On May 11, we started at the Santa Monica Pier. My second run of the trip, on day two, was one of my favorites. I started out on Highway 2 in Los Angeles, where the Angeles Crest 100 Mile Endurance Race starts. That race was one of the more well-known events in the country, and it meant about as much to me as any race. This place was important to me, as it reminded me of some of my very first hundred-mile races, where I got my start and became Catra Corbett. These are the races that made me the strong and fierce woman I am today.

While out there, I thought about how cool it was that I was now running across the country with this team, possibly helping others overcome their own addictions. Tears came to my eyes.

Near the end of my run was a preview of what we'd be facing running through the US in the summer on blacktop road. As we approached Arizona and the desert, I could feel the heat peeling off the road and surrounding my face. This was going to be a hot trip. I was glad to be at the end of the run, but I knew I had many more to go.

As we made our way into Arizona, on day three, a bunch of my friends came out to cheer us on. One of them was clean and sober again. The last time I saw him, a few months prior, he was drunk at my friend's house. He got back on track and shared his story about how he accomplished this as he ran with us. He simply told himself he needed himself in. He brought a friend who was in active recovery, meaning he'd only been sober for a few weeks, but he was doing well. They brought a third friend because they suspected that he needed help and were hoping he would seek it after being around those two for the weekend and running with us.

On day five, we made our way into New Mexico, and I was initially excited to be running through a state that had Roswell, a city known for aliens. Roswell was exactly the kind of weird shit that I loved, the Goth part of me that stayed around after my addiction.

But New Mexico was where I realized that America was full of all kinds of people and that we would be dealing with all kinds of sketchy situations, or exactly the kind of thing you see as an addict.

A couple of times we would have dogs approach us, running out of houses that looked abandoned in the middle of nowhere, and some of them were these big ass dogs that looked like they could swallow you in one gulp. But they would usually run off with a squirt of pepper spray.

It was the people who were scary. At one point, I was running along a highway that led to Roswell when a mini-van pulled up with two guys inside. Our crew van had gone up ahead. They reeked and looked like they had been up for days. I recognized that look from the people I used to hang with all the time. They were clearly meth addicts.

"Are you running by yourself?" they asked, still driving alongside me.

"Nope," I said, remembering those hikers on the trail who told me to never say I was alone. "I'm running with a team." I told them about our mission. Most people always seemed inspired when we talked to them about our goal; not these two guys.

"We don't see anyone with you," one answered.

I began to think about how I was going to get away if they pulled over when I looked up and saw our van steaming back down the road. Those guys immediately gunned it out of there.

Yet for every strange, sketchy situation, there seemed to be a couple encounters every day that made me smile through my run. Just a couple hours after those guys, I met a mother who drove all the way from Colorado to meet us in New Mexico just to have us talk to her boys about the repercussions of using drugs. She had no other answers and was losing hope. Her sons listened to all our stories and seemed inspired. Several months later, we'd hear that they were all doing well.

These meetings acted as reminders of the purpose of our trip, and they didn't just come from strangers. As I was running through New Mexico, a good friend of mine who had run many ultramarathons heard about our trip sent me an email that she was thinking about suicide. She has a chronic disease and just didn't want to go on suffering. She had a young son who needed her, but she thought she would be better to him dead. If she successfully attempted suicide with assistance, she would leave her son in a better place.

She was depressed about her divorce and the struggle she faced every day because of the limitations of her illness. I messaged her and told her that she wasn't allowed to do that. She was too much of a role model for others and for her son and that she has to live.

She messaged me back and thanked me for leading her out of her dark moment.

She just had to live each day. She just had to get by with a little help from her friends.

We made it to Roswell, and I really wanted to see the aliens. The town was rad. There were statues of aliens everywhere, and I loved walking through all the kinky stores. Charlie, who was my running partner for the moment, and I talked to a woman who believed she saw an alien once. She said she was passing by an open field when she saw a flash of light and suddenly she was somewhere else, with figures with large heads looking over her. Then she woke up, she said, disheveled in her bed.

As the first week wound up, we would get some bad news. On our way to Texas, Chris tore his Achilles tendon and would obviously not be able to run any longer.

We were each now going to have to make up about another hour a day. It doesn't sound like a lot, but when you had the load we were running, it would be pretty brutal. It could be the difference between some of us making it all the way.

But as it turns out, a friend of mine named Phil Nimmo was going to meet us once we got to the other side of Texas. Phil was also an ultrarunner. He was also sort of my boyfriend, though—as you would expect by now, it's complicated.

"Hey Charlie," I said. "What about Phil?"

In 2015, I was invited to help crew and pace a runner at Badwater that year. He was Phil, and at the time, he was new to ultrarunning. The only thing I knew about him was that they told me he was the guy to contact when I had plans to run a triple dare on the Tahoe Rim Trail, meaning three laps around the seventy-two-mile lake there. There was only one other person who had done that before: him.

I didn't end up contacting him, opting to do a double dare, or two laps, instead. The next time his name came up was in relation to crewing him at Badwater.

I thought it would be awesome to be on his crew. You have to support each other in this ultra community we have, and that meant sometimes doing the grunt work of crewing rather than the fun part of running across the finish line.

I reached out, and we got to know each other a bit through emails, and even though his crew was not organized, we got along pretty well. We decided we would meet at a few more races.

In January, we met at the Coldwater Rumble 100, and there we started talking about doing something fun together in the Sierra Nevadas in the spring. When spring came, I gave him a tour of the Sierras and we did some runs together out there. We got along well, and he asked me if I would be on his crew for Badwater for the second time, and I said that was fine, if I could be his crew chief. He agreed.

After being in California for a couple of races, Phil decided that he loved California so much that he wanted to leave Texas to live here. The attraction of California wasn't me yet—it was complicated—but completely the allure of Cali ultrarunning.

As we passed through on the Icebreaker. Phil was still living in Texas, currently entrenched in the process of selling his house. He postponed that process to help out a friend and join our team. Phil was good that way, always willing to lend a helping hand. It was a huge lift for our team to have him come out to save us. Although never having had struggled with the extent of addiction that most of us had—he had had some eating issues and alcohol problems years ago—he fully supported our mission.

The first night Phil joined us, on day eight, it was a stormy night, and it was my turn to go run. If you'll remember, I am freaked out by thunder and lightning. Running in it, I was petrified. Lightning boomed all around us, and Phil had to wonder what he was getting into when I asked him if, that night, he could just keep running after his shift was over.

He did, no questions asked.

Phil's good that way.

On top of the millions of miles already on my legs, I trained specifically for this event. A couple of weeks before starting, I had picked a week and ran a marathon every day, on the road, to get used to the grind.

By the end of the first week, we began to adjust to the grind. Our legs no longer felt drained after we finished a run. But the grind was more than just the running. Besides running every sixteen hours or so, we had to change clothes, change out the drivers and the crew, and sometimes drive ahead to the next town to be ready to start another leg. Plus we still had to eat, do laundry, and shower every once in a while. We weren't sleeping more than a few hours every night.

As we continued to make our way through Texas, the state introduced us to a new challenge, and it would be tougher than the many miles we had to knock off. Texas is not only hot—boiling hot—it is humid.

California, where I live, as well as Arizona and New Mexico were hot, but they had dry air, the kind of air I was used to running in. But Texas, and the rest of the southern states, were humid, even wet.

Once I actually ran, rather than think about the huge task ahead of me, I could break it down into manageable chunks of effort. Phil and I would work out a system where we would each do three and a half hours each for our first run, and then a shorter run for our second. It was doable.

The only problem to our perfect system? I was soaked after my first run. I'd be dripping wet. I wasn't used to this at all.

"What the fuck is this?" I screeched as I finished my third day of running through Texas, which I found to be a big, hot, miserable state. I felt like I'd just jumped in a pool. I had to strip down and get into my second outfit just to ride in the RV. When Phil was done with his first shift, I'd run my second, and come back soaking wet again, even though

I'd run less than an hour. I'd have to change again just to sleep, and then do it all over again the next day. We went through laundry like teenagers. We stunk like them too.

At the end of our second week, we were in the Deep South, and I was not used to the Deep South, and the people who lived there were not used to me. I ran through a lot of tiny towns, with the air feeling like a swamp, and I began to count all the strange looks I got. People just stared at me as I ran by their front porches.

In fairness to them, there weren't many tattooed people running through the heat of the day with their piercings clinking around their faces and their pink hair tied into a ponytail.

Because I was the Dirt Diva, there were people who knew me and wanted to run with me. And yet, I wasn't the one who gained fame as the trip went on. Most people who came out didn't want to see me. They wanted to see the "running wiener dog." They wanted to see TruMan. More and more people stopped us so they could see the ultrarunning dog. People were fascinated with the fact that this little dog on tiny legs could run so far, but I'd like to think it was his story that touched people. TruMan came from a bad situation, and people began to take strength in his story.

TruMan really blossomed on this trip. He was with strangers all day, usually, because I was out running, and he slept in all these unknown hotel rooms at night. He grew more and more comfortable with the strange surroundings. This was huge for the little dog who wouldn't come out from behind the couch when I first got him. Now he was fine riding in a strange car with stranger people and hearing new sounds all the time. He was no longer afraid of new experiences in the world. He was embracing them.

As proof, TruMan finally got the courage to bark when he didn't recognize someone. With his newfound confidence, he finally felt like he could alert me and even protect me from people. It was pretty cool that he became that confident. Apparently all that fame went to his head.

Our little group had a huge following that only seemed to get bigger every day. As the word about us bounded around the South, we had people come out wanting to run with us every single day, even if it was at 2 a.m. It filled my heart with joy and brought tears to my eyes. Almost every person who came out wanted to share their story with us.

People, in fact, wanted to run with us especially if it was 2 a.m. because that seemed to be the only part of the day that didn't threaten to burn you if you ran for too long. On day 15, in Mississippi, the heat was so bad that Phil, who lives in Texas and was training for Badwater, the hottest ultramarathon in the country, nearly passed out and had to stop. I had to take over for him. As soon as I left the comfort of the RV, I felt as if my skin was melting.

A man who looked to be in his fifties drove by slowly on the road, staring at me as he passed. I tried to laugh it off. *This was the South, not California*, I thought. He, like many in the South, wasn't used to seeing crazy people like me.

The second time he drove past me, I got a little worried. He rolled down his window, and I looked up at my van, hoping they would come back. I looked for a rope on his dashboard.

"Lady, it's hot out here," he said. "I just want to give you some water."

He didn't know why I was running, but he wanted to share something with me. It was so sweet. When I explained our mission, after I gratefully chugged the water, he said one of his sons was a drug addict.

We began our last week of running, on day 18, in South Carolina. That night, Phil was almost hit by a car.

It was 11 p.m., and I was filling his water and trying to find him some food. We were near a bar, waiting for Phil to catch us, and all of a sudden, I heard Phil in the distance yelling at this guy to fuck off. When I looked up, startled, I saw Phil flying off the road.

South Carolina, at least where we were running, didn't have any shoulders on its highways, and as Phil was running along, a car came right at him. Phil had to jump in some weeds and rolled down a small hill. I thought he'd been hit.

We were running out of the van in the black night, following the sound of Phil's cussing, when the car whipped around and started speeding for us.

Phil had a handheld bottle, and to get the driver's attention, just before he dove into the weeds, he threw it at the car's windshield. The bottle cracked off the windshield and broke it.

Both the driver and Phil began screaming at each other, and I began to worry if the driver had a gun. One of our drivers was ex-military, and he had a gun too. I was almost relieved when the four cop cars showed up, lights blaring. When the officers came out, I knew we were in trouble.

"What were you doing on the road this late at night?" one of the officers asked Phil.

They began to call the driver by his name.

Shit.

Well, the question was fair, but I was pissed, and I answered that it was because there was no fucking shoulder on the road. We were trying to run for mental health awareness. The officer answered that we didn't seem very stable. That pissed me off even more. They began to threaten to throw Phil in jail.

Phil, however, is a civil, calm person. He apologized for the mirror, and he said he would pay for it. This calmed the situation right away. He got the guy's email address. The cops then escorted us out of the county.

As a side note, Phil did email the guy, and when we got home from the run, he mailed him the check to repair the windshield with a note as to why were out there running late at night.

To this day, that check had not been cashed.

The end approached, and on day 22, on my first shift through Virginia, our last state, even though I was glad we were almost done, I was also sorry to have this journey end. Our collective email inbox, which we checked several times a day on the road, filled with messages every day from people who wanted to come meet us.

Everyone had a story, and on one of my last runs of the trip, I thought about some of the ones that I still think about on my training runs today. Some of these stories came from the South, a place where I felt at first I didn't understand the people, and they didn't understand me. In Arkansas, a woman told me she suffered from sexual abuse and turned to drugs to mask the shame and the pain, much like I did. She came to accept who she was and what had happened to her after hearing about the cause of our run. She changed her life and got off the drugs. A year later, in 2017, she ran her first hundred-miler.

In Georgia, a guy who ran with us said he had been in prison for five years for robbing a bank to pay for drugs. He got sober in prison and was released a couple years ago. He struggled with his desire to do drugs when he was released, so he turned to running. He heard about our group through his running club. Ultrarunning is now his life, much like it is for mine.

In Virginia, on day 23, we finished at the Mental Health America conference. The non-profit is one of the leading organizations in addressing the needs of those with mental illness.

They announced each one of us, and we ran through the crowd and up on the stage. When they announced my name and TruMan's name, I raised him up over my head, and I teared up because I realized I had been through so much shit to get up on that stage. We all had. All these people fought with me, for me, and for themselves.

I'm still fighting.

Chapter Twenty-Two

Another Year, Thanks to Running

Sometime in the early nineties—I was on drugs so I don't exactly remember—I'd been awake for three or four days straight. I'd been clubbing and was coming off a binge. I was in the burn stage, and I was watching TV and wishing for it to be over.

A show where people were running caught my eye on the TV. Whenever I saw someone running on TV, it reminded me of watching Western States with my father, so I stopped on the channel. It was a story about the Badwater race, a 135-mile jaunt through Death Valley, in the hottest part of the summer in the hottest part of the country. *These people were crazy*, I thought.

I also remember being out the next night, on meth again, in the club, and talking to my friends about it. Of course because everyone was on drugs, everyone's reaction was "Whoa, those people are really whacked out."

The reality is we were the whacked out ones. I learned that many years later. Those runners were the normal ones. Sort of normal, anyway.

From that point on, it was always in the back of my head that I wanted to run Badwater, but I always came up with excuses not to. I wasn't a road runner or I couldn't afford it, or something like that. But one of the main reasons was even though I said I really wanted to do it, I *didn't* really want to do it.

The race came up in discussion for the first time in my running career in 2004, when Crazy Linda was running it for the second time. She asked me to be on her crew.

I knew what the race entailed. I did some sauna training just to pace her. I was doing a lot of ultras by this point, and I'd seen a lot of shit. But Badwater was its own special kind of shit.

Badwater might be the toughest ultramarathon in the country. You have to be trained not only to run a hundred miles but to withstand temperatures of well over 100 degrees, which is the real challenge. All the running takes place on asphalt, and in the heat of the day, runners' lost their shoes because they were melting on the surface.

I was trained to run in that furnace, and I prided myself on being able to run in the heat, yet I struggled. Other seemed to be destroyed by it. It was the kind of event that could turn even those who had finished many hundred-milers into puddles of sweat, puke, and tears.

Throughout the race, I watched Linda go through these incredible ups and downs. She would cry and laugh, and it was amazing to me how she would essentially fall down and pick herself up again. This race destroyed people, but not her.

These people really are crazy, I thought to myself. Maybe my old self was right. But we got through it, and when Linda asked me back to crew her during her third Badwater, I came back, and it was fun once again to watch. It was fun to be a part of that. I kind of wanted to do it on my own.

In 2009, I got accepted into the Badwater race and got involved with a Badwater race crew, and things went wrong from the start. It just didn't feel right. There was intense drama going on between the crew leaders and it just seemed like bad karma to be a part of that, and so I dropped out a month before the start.

I didn't need Badwater. I had all my other hundreds that I loved. There were always things to do.

So Badwater was not a priority, but once again, it came back to me. It is how Phil and I became friends. When I crewed him, I learned a lot about what not to do. I'd been on a lot of organized crews, and this was the complete opposite. Other crew members put Phil's food on ice, and the food got soggy because ice tends to melt when it's 115 degrees. There also wasn't a lot of food to begin with. Phil had to eat a lot of pickles because eventually that's all we had. But he did finish. And the next year, Phil asked me to crew again, and after I said I needed to be crew chief, he agreed to that, and I figured out this race even more.

I was in my fifties when I finally decided to run it for myself.

When I got into Badwater through the lottery in 2017, I knew I'd have to train for the heat as well as the miles.

I started by wearing three layers of clothing while running, a Gore-Tex jacket, a hat, and a parka in the heat of the day in the spring in California.

I also trained by sitting in a sauna for up to an hour. I would just sit there and sweat.

Also to prepare, I ran the Kokopelli 150 Stage Race from Grand Junction, Colorado, through a desert to Moab, Utah. Stages races were unusual, but they had their advantages. You didn't, for instance, have to run all 150 miles of it at one chunk. You ran six days, and every day, there was a set amount to run. Stage One was twenty miles. But it was also through remote desert, and every runner was responsible for herself, with only a handful of aid stations to bail you out. Despite all the work I did to get used to the heat, in the second day during a thirty-nine-mile stage through the desert, I had to stop at mile thirty-three. I struggled a lot, and I felt demoralized. The heat is never a joke, but I'd never let it stop me, and I'd trained for it even beyond my own ability to deal with the heat. In a way, it was understandable, given that I was running through the desert. But then again, a question loomed in my head.

How was I going to do Badwater?

My answer, besides my own preparation and toughness, was in my crew.

During the race, my crew refilled my bottles, took care of my food, and made sure I had enough of both. They paced me. They encouraged me. When I got hot, they fanned me to cool me off. When I was sore— and I got sore—they massaged out the pain.

They also kept me distracted by telling stories. You find out all about other people's relationships, if they're being cheated on or if they're cheating, and if they're considering a divorce. You find out their health problems. You find all about their pasts before running helped them get over whatever it was haunting them. You act as each other's therapists out there a lot of the time. I've told people many things to many people out there that I've never told anyone else.

As I stood there, waiting for the start, I knew that I had a hot, uncertain and painful forty-two hours ahead of me. We were waiting for the national anthem to get us off, and Chris, the race director, was having trouble with his recording. A member of my crew offered to sing and everyone there started singing with her.

The race went off. Eventually, as Badwater will, it got really hot after a nice night and a spell when it even started raining. My crew kept wetting me down, icing down my legs, and easing food and drink in me. They were an amazing crew.

One of the hardest things about giving up drugs, if not the hardest, is the fact that you don't just have to give up the drugs. You have to give up your community. That, in a way, is giving up your life. You have to give up your friends and your places you go and, of course, the things you loved to do together.

I was ready to do that when I quit. None of those things had the same appeal any longer. And yet it was still hard to do that. I had to find a way out. I found it through running, and eventually, I found a new community.

So I did not trade one addiction for another. I traded one community for another.

Everyone in the ultra community is like family, even those I've barely met. When they try to shake my hand, I won't let them. I give them a hug. I feel that close to someone who runs, and especially to someone who runs ultras.

When you're having a rough day, they're the ones who get to the finish.

When you're having a rough month, they're the ones who get you to the next race.

When you're having a rough year, they're the ones who get you through to the next one.

Over the years, they have sent me flowers, paid my airfare with points, shared rooms with me the night before a race, fed me, paced me, given me extra gear, messaged me, texted me, and called me and been my friends. They made me who I am. They made me Catra Corbett.

I finally finished Badwater in just under forty-three hours.

I could not have done it without all of them.

Inspired by an acquaintance, I decided that when I turned forty, I thought I would run an hour for every year I was alive. Some runners will go a mile for every year they're alive, but I wanted to do something a little more epic.

I did it along the Ohlone Wilderness Trail, and of course my friends came out, and it was a lot of fun. Honestly, forty hours was not that big of a deal at that point. My friends asked me if I was going to do it next year.

Uh, well, I guess so.

So I did do it every year, and my plan was to do it until I turned fifty. Then, because fifty is such a milestone, I thought I wouldn't have to do it anymore.

I turned fifty, and I ran for fifty hours.

It is not as bad as you might think. I raise money for a cause each time. That keeps me going. I make it a low key thing, so if I want to nap, I will nap, and if I want to get something to eat or get a coffee at Starbucks, I'll do that. My friends come out, and I give them swag bags and treats and drinks, and it's really fun.

While I really wanted to be done at year fifty, and yet, the next year I did fifty-one hours. Then I did fifty-two hours. In 2018, I'll do fifty-three.

Why do I continue to do it? Well, I don't think to set limits on myself. Sometimes you may not want to get out there, but you just keep going and trudging along and doing the best you can. I just do it and don't think about it. That's how I get through a tough run. That's how you get through life.

I don't have any regrets about my past. Everything in your life has to happen the way it happened in order to be who you are in your life. I had to be a drug addict to become an ultrarunner. I had to find a passion in order to overcome my addiction.

Even the death of my parents, which continues to break my heart, helped me become who I am today. My dad, in his small ways, helped put ultrarunning in my head, from the time he had me watch a few minutes of the Western States 100 with him. When she died, my mother left me money to enter those races. Without that I'm not sure if I would have found a love for Yosemite, since I was looking for a place to heal. I would like them to be here now, of course, and I wish my father could be around to see what I've done. But I'm not sure I would be the same person if he was.

My yearly run is a reminder of my own rebirth. I love the reminder that I'm another year older, mainly because of running.

There are many things I think about when I remember my run across America. It changed my life. It made me want to be a better person. We all go through struggles, but I think about the hundreds of people we met along the way who shared their story about their own problems and struggles and issues. They were struggling to be a better person every day. That made me want to be that person as well. I have to keep trudging for them.

But I also think about the very beginning of the race, when I got to run through Hollywood, California. I was in that area a lot when I was a Goth. More than twenty years ago, I was doing meth in those areas. Now, I thought, I was running through these areas, clean and sober, for a purpose: fighting against addiction. I made myself a new life. I hope others can do the same by following my example.

I still think about my sister when I'm alone on a run. She is one of the many people from my life who are now gone who run the trails with me in my heart. I think about my father, who loved to run. I think about my mother, whose determination carries me past the agony of the worst of what running can bring. I think about Suzanne, who showed me how tough someone could be. I think about Rocky and all those dogs that showed me how being in a tough situation doesn't mean you have to be in that situation forever.

I need my running community. All of it. But when I don't have pacers, I have those people by my side.

I had another birthday challenge the year I turned forty-eight. I thought I would run for forty-eight days straight. Well, I made it to day forty-nine, and I just kept going. I just kept trudging along. I'm now approaching my fifty-third birthday, and I've run every day since I was forty-eight.

I just never stopped.
After all, I am an ultrarunner.

Author's Note

My First Ultramarathon
by Dan England

When I flew out in 2013 to write a long story for *SBNation* about ultra-running, addiction, and Catra, I knew, deep down, that I wanted to be an ultrarunner.

I just didn't know how to do it.

When I was out there, I ran Mission Peak, the same mountain Catra has run more than four thousand times, and I loved how it reminded me of my past life.

I was a mountaineer many years ago. I loved hiking in beautiful, remote areas in Colorado, and I loved the challenge of getting to those places both by car and by foot. I invested many hours of sweat and pain and some blood in those spots. I devoted my life to them, even moving out to Greeley in 1999 just so I could be closer to the peaks.

I switched to running after I climbed all fifty-four of the fourteen-thousand-foot peaks in Colorado, what we call the 14ers. I had to find a new challenge after my children were born. The time the peaks took away from my kids was mostly unacceptable, and putting my life at risk seemed foolish at best and selfish at worst.

Running, for many years, did provide that challenge, but I missed the trails, and after many years, I burned out of running as hard as I could. I desperately wanted to find my way back to my first love.

When I went out with Catra to a race where she "only" ran a 50K that weekend, I was, of course, inspired by the many who were running a hundred miles in a stifling heat that made me miserable even sitting in a chair. But I also discovered something: ultrarunning was possible.

There were people at the race with all kinds of shapes, from pears to princes, and most of them looked, well, normal. They just had a determination that you don't see in most people. That's what separated them from the crowd.

I left that race newly inspired and before I flew home, the next morning, I went out to the Big Basin State Park, where giant redwoods loomed over trails, and ran thirteen miles. My life as an ultrarunner started that day.

What follows is a description of my first ultramarathon. If there is any way to thank Catra for showing me another life, this is it.

"Why do we do this? You hear, all the time, 'because it's fun.' But we don't do it for that. We do it because it's hard."—Fred Abramowitz

At 4 a.m., the inky-black mountain air hung with frost, and my brain tried one desperate, last-ditch attempt at self-preservation.

You didn't sleep much, part of it whispered to me, *and this warm bed feels so comfy.*

Fred Abramowitz, Run Rabbit Run's race director, said this would happen. The night before, after warning us about wrong turns that led us far from home, ornery moose, and the aid station cutoffs, he told us there was a part of our brain that would try to convince us to quit.

This part was a small lizard that crawled from the ocean, Abramowitz said at the meeting, and found the first rock it could crawl under. It's the part that whimpers at the first sign of pain. It's the part that tells you to eat the whole half gallon of ice cream.

"Promise me you won't listen to that part tomorrow," he said to us.

The thing is, the Lizard is hard to ignore. At 4 a.m., the Lizard was doing its best to convince me to stay in bed. I was about to try to run fifty miles. I was forty-four years old and had never run that far before.

I'd never even run a 50K, let alone fifty miles. And Run Rabbit Run was one of the hardest fifty-milers in the country, a race that hovered around ten thousand feet at times and made you climb more than nine thousand feet, essentially three 14ers. It was going to hurt.

Abramowitz said that too.

"You could just walk around downtown and play Pokémon Go," the Lizard whispered, "and no one would blame you for that. Spend the day with your family. Go see Fish Creek Falls."

I got the coffee going, peed, and dove back into bed. Maybe the Lizard was right. I honestly didn't know if I could finish. I'd never felt that about a race, even races that went up Mount Evans or Pikes Peak or at one of my five marathons. Even with a forecast that promised perfect weather, the fact that I survived the training without getting hurt and a chance to see Steamboat and one of the prettiest places on Earth, I didn't know if I could run that far or fast enough to make the fifteen-hour cutoff.

I've climbed all the 14ers and ran all those races above and completed many half marathons. I've run fast enough to make the first few waves of the Boulder Bolder. But I am not an elite athlete. Most people in good condition could do what I do, with the right experience and training, and many could do it better.

The coffee smelled good. I sighed and pushed the covers away.

This was not a sure thing. How many times would I attempt something like that in my adult life? I wanted to see if it was possible.

I threw on my shorts and top before I changed my mind and began to struggle to pull on my compression calf sleeves.

"Seriously, dude," the Lizard whined. "Don't do this."

"Shut up," I said back.

At 6 a.m., a close friend of mine, Michael Mock, and I waited in the back of the pack for the "Star-Spangled Banner" or a gun or some pounding pump-up music from One Direction, but when the 194 headlamps started bobbing toward the start, I realized, once again, this was not a

Rock 'n' Roll Half Marathon. We had a 3,700-foot climb ahead of us, a tough six-mile start, and Abramowitz seemed to know we couldn't spend an ounce of energy whooping it up.

I thought about running, but Mock, who completed the Mount Hood 50 earlier that year, cautioned me about going out too hard, and I nodded in agreement. I learned early on in my training that running up hills saved you a few minutes, but you paid dearly in spent energy for that extra time.

Those few minutes were indeed important in a half marathon, possibly the difference between a PR and any other race, but in an ultra, those extra minutes are a sneeze and a cough. "Save your strength," Mock told me. The Lizard would have agreed, but he was pouting.

I started chirping about a quarter mile up Mount Werner. Sometimes I'm quiet, sometimes not, but I'm rarely chatty. Mock smirked as he breathed with his Iowa lungs through the thin air. I tried to enjoy the energy that came from the relief of finally getting to try something that had been in my head for almost a year.

A year ago, as I flew down the Poudre Canyon in the Equinox Half Marathon, I realized that I hated running. I was sick of feeling sick and full of fire and bile as I gasped my way to another finish. I ran another half, the Golden Leaf in Aspen, a week later, dreading it but not wanting to waste the entry fee.

Aspen's hard but beautiful trails gave me an excuse to take it easy. I just wanted to finish, and I loved every second of it. I wanted a race like that one, with a goal to finish, only at a distance that would push me. I'd done a marathon, and a 50K was only six miles longer. A fifty-miler seemed perfect. It was crazy, but not inconceivable, like a hundred-miler was.

I picked Run Rabbit Run because it was one of the most prestigious ultramarathons in Colorado. The race gives away as much money as any other ultra in the country, and that draws a nice crowd. It was also beautiful and had a good reputation as a well-run, well-respected race.

But I mostly picked it because Steamboat was one of the few places in Colorado I had yet to see. I entered it early and became one of the most annoying people on the planet. Even my running friends who loved nothing more than racing every weekend were sick of hearing about my training or my excitement or, most of all, my fears about finishing.

Six miles up, in just under two hours, I summited Werner, with Mock close behind. I could tell he was struggling, and I knew it was time to say goodbye. *I'll see you out there*, I whispered to him and took off.

Five minutes later, my elation at summiting was blitzed by my first dark moment of the race.

Abramowitz warned us about those, too. The enormity of the race hit me. I had just climbed a mountain, was really feeling it, and I had forty-four miles to go. Forty-four! I had hoped to make it to the turn-around point, just under twenty-six miles, in six and a half hours. I'd need to start running now, or else I wasn't going to make it, and I didn't feel like running.

The Lizard chuckled. "See? I told you," he said. I shooed him from my mind and scanned the runners for a buddy. Mark, a fifty-some-year-old from Longmont, trailed right behind me, and I started our new relationship with the easy ice-breaker: "Is this your first?" It was. We repeated some small talk that we'd exchanged up the mountain, as I forgot we'd already talked a bit—the altitude will do that to you—and we started running. I told him, several times, to pass me if I was holding him up, but he finally told me to stop asking. A third voice filtered out of the woods, this one belonging to Rachel, a thirty-something female also in her first. Both were relatively normal people looking for a new challenge, like me, although I also got the sense that Mark had a wife who had completed Ironman events, so he was looking for something of his own, and Rachel was a counselor for students and needed to burn off the tension she felt from their hard lives.

We chatted for the next seventeen miles, which made me forget that we were running up and down on trails. Time few by, and soon we celebrated at Long Lake and the fact that we had just nearly completed a half marathon. We didn't think about the fact that we had three more to go.

When I entered Run Rabbit Run, I relied on the book *Relentless Forward Progress* by Byron Powell, an ultramarathoner who ran the website "I Run Far," a highly respected site that followed some of the best races in the world, some advice from Catra Corbett (hi Catra!) and my own instincts for a training plan. I also relied on Pokémon Go. I'll get to that in a bit.

I pieced together a plan that I hoped would allow me to stay married—I have a patient wife and three kids, including nine-year-old twins—stay healthy and stay focused. Powell had a plan that allowed you to train for a fifty-miler on less than fifty miles a week. The long runs, he wrote, mattered far more than the weekday ones.

After a few months, I did a twenty-miler through a cold, hard rain to get ready for a marathon. I ran the Greenland 25K in a blizzard, and then, a week later, I did the Revel marathon down Mount Charleston in May in Vegas and felt good.

I leaned on back-to-back long runs until the race approached, and I then planned on three runs of five to six hours. I bought a hydration backpack and hit trails such as Horsetooth Mountain in Fort Collins and Devil's Backbone in Loveland. My first big run was in Rocky Mountain National Park, for twenty miles and five thousand feet of elevation gain, and I felt elated but exhausted afterward. My next big run was during our family vacation, when I ran down the Grand Canyon to the Colorado River and back, nine thousand feet up and down. I cramped up and could barely walk by the time I got back to our cabin, an hour later than my family expected. I was so out of it for an hour after that that my oldest, my son, Jayden, asked "Mommy, is Daddy going to die?"

All these training runs reminded me how to suffer. There's all kinds of things you need to learn before an ultra—how to eat, how to drink, how to pace yourself—but mostly, you just need to learn how to run when you're in pain and exhausted and hot or cold.

My last long run, a twenty-seven-miler over Devil's, went well, but it didn't help much with the anxiety I felt about running fifty miles. At this point, both Powell and some experienced ultrarunners insisted that I was probably ready. It seemed weird to me that running twenty-seven meant I could run fifty. In fact, it made no sense at all.

At mile twenty-two, there's a place, the Dumont Campground, where spectators cheer for you before you tackle Rabbit Ears Pass, the second major climb of the day and the turnaround. It's a stark reminder that you live among people, in civilization, something you honestly question in between aid stations, when you're running on trails so remote, with only shreds of blue ribbons to guide you, locales where spraining an ankle could mean you become moose food. Most of the spectators were there to hug their family members, fiercely, before allowing them back out into the wild. A new friend who was on my Ragnar Relay team a few weeks earlier gave me a hug. It was so good to see a friendly face.

When I bent down to tie my shoe, a sudden spray of kisses greeted me, and I looked through blurry eyes to see a chocolate lab wagging his butt and saying hi. I'm a dog person, and dogs somehow know this.

"That's Ranger," said one of the volunteers. "He's our therapy dog for ultrarunners."

I petted Ranger many times and soaked up the good vibes. I knew I'd need them.

The hill up Rabbit Ears was not very steep, but it was too steep to run. As I worked my way up, the sun started to beat down on my neck, and I started to sweat for the first time that day. At mile eighteen, I've never been so happy to pee in my life because it meant I was actually drinking enough.

Rabbit Ears turned into a mountain, almost to the point where I couldn't even walk straight. I focused on the exchanges of encouragement between the (many) faster runners and me as we passed each other. And then, suddenly, I was at the top.

A rush of energy hit me. The cold wind vaporized my sweaty skin and left me shivering. I then realized that every step I took from then on would bring me home. I looked at my watch. 6:40. That wasn't fast, but it gave me a really good shot to finish. And I would get to see some friends, both new and old, on the way down.

I high-fived Mark and Rachel and started flying down the hill. I felt awesome. Honestly, it probably wasn't smart to run that hard, but this is why you train. You don't train just to finish a race. You train for the moments when you feel invincible. It makes me sad that most people don't experience these moments the way I do in a race. It's these moments that get me through life.

I ran into Mike back near the campground, and he was still struggling but hanging in there. I hugged him and tried to encourage him but didn't stay long.

There is a moment in every race when it gets harder than you'd like. Only a few miles after I celebrated the fact that I felt good and had run farther than I ever had in my life, the race started to turn.

At the next aid station, after changing my socks with Rachel by my side and Mark eating some chips, I chugged some Gatorade. I was really thirsty. I also took a HOTSHOT, an anti-cramping drink, because I'd had trouble with that before and felt some warning signs, such as my left hamstring seizing up as I put on my shoe again.

My stomach was already angry at me before I left the aid station.

Only the best ultrarunners actually run the whole race. You run enough to give yourself a good cushion for walking. At mile thirty-five, my stomach began to bother me, and I realized that there would be a point where I'd have to accept the fact that I wouldn't be running much the rest of the race. I had given myself that cushion. I hoped it was enough.

As I continued to hike more and more, I found myself grateful for Pokémon Go.

I began to walk at night, for an hour or so, in spots where the cartoon critters were supposed to hang out. I got into the game a little bit too much because I tend to be that way, and I found myself walking up to fifteen miles a week, chasing down Pokémon in parks, through downtown Greeley, and in and out of our two college campuses.

The walking helped me recover from the long runs, and it kept me on my feet.

Thank you, Snorlax.

The nausea reached a crescendo as I climbed up a small incline, and then the despair hit me as I realized what was going to happen. My stomach clenched. I retched. I leaned over and heaved. Nothing came out. I heaved and choked, and my stomach recoiled and tried again, and nothing came out again, save for my whimpers of pain.

I tried to gasp for air in between the convulsions.

Then it was over, and I started to breathe again. At mile forty-one, with our final aid station up Mount Werner still two hours away, my stomach ruled the run.

Just keep moving, I told myself.

I traded places with Mark off and on the trail, but we didn't say much to each other except weak hellos when we did approach. Rachel was long gone, eventually finishing in under thirteen hours. I stuck in my headphones and cranked up my metal. I honestly don't know how people do hard, dark things without metal to get them through them. Taylor Swift just doesn't do it in those moments.

I caught a first glimpse of Werner with mixed emotions. I knew if I could get there, the hard part was way over. But the mountain looked far away, just a speck against the sky, which already seemed to be losing light.

No way we have to climb all that, I thought.

We did. I would imagine that last fifteen hundred feet probably cost a good portion of the people the race. Indeed, Mike climbed it but missed the cutoff to the last aid station by eleven minutes.

Races like this one can carry you for years during some dark moments. As I hinted at earlier, even we normal folks seem to have another reason to run crazy stuff like this. I lost a piece of my self-esteem after junior high school, when I was bullied, and things like this help replace it. Racing is enough to stop depression and soften my anxiety.

But man, that last thousand feet were tough. I topped out at the last Mount Werner aid station, cried a bit, which is unlike me, and yet another wonderful volunteer dressed me like a toddler, throwing my layers on me and offered me some much-needed advice on how to drink fluids on an evil stomach (sip water, slowly). He got me going with something that made me cry again.

"You've got two and a half hours to do less than six miles," he said and smiled. "Enjoy your walk down."

One of my running partners met me with five miles to go. I still had to walk nearly four thousand feet down. But I knew the hard part was over.

It was dark near the end, so dark that I couldn't really see, even with a headlamp. My kids hoped to run me in but missed me, and I crossed the line forty-five minutes before the cutoff, as one of the last ten people among the 160 or so who finished. I saw friends and soaked up their congratulations, both on Facebook and in person, and then went back to the hotel, where we went in the hot tub. Then I showered and went to bed for a hard night of achy sleep.

The next morning, I got up to hit the bathroom, winced, and went back to bed before we went to Steamboat's hot springs pool later that day. That night I would play Pokémon Go around downtown Steamboat.

When we left the day after that, on a Monday, I thought about getting up to run. The Lizard poked his head out from under the rock.

"You need to rest," he said.

Sometimes the Lizard is right. I walked instead, for a couple miles. You do need a break. I was looking forward to a week or two off from running, and a whole lot of ice cream, before I started ignoring him again.

Acknowledgments

When I set out to write a book, I didn't realize how difficult it would be. Going back and reliving your past takes a lot of guts.

It takes a lot of time and energy to do this. And I appreciate everyone who inspired me to do this and supported me through the process. I want to thank my parents who are no longer with me.

My mom and dad have inspired me and shaped me into who I am today. Without them I wouldn't be here and this book would not be possible. To all my friends out there who encourage me to write a book. They often would say to me, "you have the best stories." Thank you all.

Finally, some of my crazy life stories are told here. For Phil my adventuring partner and partner in life thanks for putting up with me through the whole process of writing this book ,and being there to support me and helping me when I needed help during these times. I want to thank TruMan, my faithful four-legged companion for the last six years who is gotten me through so many dark times and so many happy times. He has inspired me so much more than any human ever has. He has made me a better person and taught me to push harder and to be runstoppable.

Thanks Dan England for believing in me and helping me get my story out there. It wasn't easy, I know, and it took a lot of hard work but through this we got it done together.

I'm excited to inspire all of you to push past what you think is actually possible. You don't have to be a runner to be inspired; you just have to want to get out and do better in life.

Life is too short to sit around, so I encourage you all to get out and find your passion in life and do makes you happy. Live life, love life.

I want to add for all the people who suffer from addiction and mental health issues there is always help and don't be afraid to ask for it. The first step is always the hardest part. But once you get help, you too can be amazing.